# The Anti-Inflammatory Diet

*Easy Recipes for Beginners Who Want to Feel Better Every Day (with Pictures)*

*Lily Serene*

## Disclaimer Notice:

Please note the information contained within this document is for educational and entertainment purposes only. All effort has been executed to present accurate, up to date, and reliable, complete information. No warranties of any kind are declared or implied. Readers acknowledge that the author is not engaging in the rendering of legal, financial, medical or professional advice. The content within this book has been derived from various sources. Please consult a licensed professional before attempting any techniques outlined in this book.

By reading this document, the reader agrees that under no circumstances is the author responsible for any losses, direct or indirect, which are incurred as a result of the use of the information contained within this document, including, but not limited to, — errors, omissions, or inaccuracie.

# Table of Content

## Chapter 5 – Main Dish Recipes ..............................122

## Chapter 6 - Side Dish Recipes ..............................157

## Chapter 7 – Dessert Recipes ...................................189

# Introduction

Hello! I'm excited to have you here at my anti-inflammatory cookbook! Welcome to this cookbook, where we will take you on a journey through the basics and mouthwatering recipes of the anti-inflammatory diet. The anti-inflammatory diet is focused to consume whole, nutrient-rich foods that can help to decrease the inflammation in your body. You can promote overall health by including these ingredients in your meals.

Inflammation is a natural and essential process that occurs in the body to protect itself when something harmful or irritating happens. It's like a response or a signal that tells the immune system to take action. When there is inflammation, the affected area may become red, swollen, warm, and painful. This response helps the body heal from injuries, fight off infections, and get rid of any harmful substances.

**For example**, if you get a cut on your finger, the area around the cut may become red and swollen. That's because your body is sending special cells and chemicals to the cut to help repair the damaged tissue and prevent infection. This is called acute inflammation, and it usually goes away once the injury is healed.

However, sometimes inflammation can become a long-term problem. This type of inflammation is called chronic inflammation, and it can happen when our body's immune system stays activated for a longer time, even when there is no injury or infection. Chronic inflammation can be caused by things like unhealthy diet, lack of exercise, stress, smoking, or exposure to toxins. It can contribute to various health issues like heart disease, diabetes, arthritis, and certain types of cancer. Taking care of your health, eating a balanced diet, getting regular exercise, managing stress, and avoiding harmful substances can help reduce inflammation and keep your body in a healthier state.

An anti-inflammatory diet can be an effective way to reduce your body's inflammation simply. When we eat certain foods, they can either increase or decrease inflammation in our bodies. An anti-inflammatory diet focuses on the consumption of foods that have lower inflammation and avoids foods that can promote inflammation.

The foods included in an anti-inflammatory diet are typically whole and nutrient-rich foods. These foods include fruits, wholegrains, vegetables, lean proteins, and healthy fats. These meals are good sources of anti-inflammatory nutrients such antioxidants, vitamins, minerals, and other helpful components.

**For example**, fruits and vegetables are full of antioxidants that can fight against harmful molecules called free radicals, which can contribute to inflammation. Omega-3 fatty acids found in fatty fish, seeds, and nuts are known for their anti-inflammatory properties. Healthy fats found in avocado and olive oils can also help to reduce inflammation.

On the other hand, an anti-inflammatory diet encourages avoiding or limiting foods that can trigger inflammation. These include highly processed foods, sugary drinks, unhealthy snacks, fried foods, and foods high in trans-fats. These types of foods can promote inflammation in the body and contribute to chronic health problems. By following an anti-inflammatory diet, you can give your body the nutrients it needs to fight inflammation and promote overall health. It's important to note that an anti-inflammatory diet is just one part of a healthy lifestyle. Regular exercise, stress management, and getting enough sleep are also important factors in reducing inflammation.

Here are some scientific research and studies that support the effectiveness of an anti-inflammatory diet:

1. A group of researchers conducted a study that was published in the Journal of Internal Medicine in 2019. They looked at information from more than 68,000 Swedish men and women to see if there was a connection between following an anti-inflammatory diet and the risk of death. According to the study, people who followed the anti-inflammatory diet had a lower risk of dying from any cause, cardiovascular diseases, and cancer, compared to those who didn't stick to the diet very well.

2. A study published in 2016 in the Journal Diabetes Care looked at how an anti-inflammatory diet affects insulin resistance and inflammatory markers in people with type 2 diabetes. The people who followed the anti-inflammatory diet for six weeks saw big improvements in how their bodies responded to insulin and had less inflammation, as shown by lower levels of IL-6 and TNF-α, compared to the group that didn't follow the diet.

3. A study published by the European Journal of Nutrition in 2020 included a randomized controlled trial which looked at how an anti-inflammatory diet affects liver enzymes, metabolic parameters, and inflammatory markers in people with non-alcoholic fatty liver disease (NAFLD). The research showed that people in the group following the anti-inflammatory diet had better results in their liver enzymes, insulin resistance, lipid profile, and inflammatory markers compared to the control group.

All these studies show that an anti-inflammatory diet might help lower the chance of getting certain diseases, make symptoms better, and have a positive effect on different health measures.

This cookbook is loaded with a variety of mouthwatering anti-inflammatory diet recipes. The recipes written in this cookbook come from different categories, such as delicious breakfasts, appetizers and snacks; to vibrant salads, main courses, side dishes, and yummy desserts. Our recipes are crafted to excite your tastebuds while providing you with a richness of essential nutrients. Our cookbook offers you easy-to-follow meal plans designed to simplify your transformation to an anti-inflammatory diet. If you still have any confusion, then say goodbye to it, and say hello to well-nourishing meals that will leave you feeling satisfied and energized.

# Chapter 1 - Anti-Inflammatory Diet

## What is Inflammation?

Inflammation is a natural immune system response that works in our body as a defense mechanism against harmful germs, bacteria, foreign invaders, viruses, etc. In certain medical conditions such as arthritis, our body's immune system malfunctions and triggers an inflammatory response even if there are no other harmful invaders in our body. In such conditions, our auto-immune system harms itself by damaging healthy tissues. There are a few signs and symptoms of inflammation including pain, swelling, heat, increase in blood flow, and loss of functions. In some cases of inflammation, there are no signs and symptoms. There are two common types of inflammation: acute inflammation and chronic inflammation:

*Acute inflammation* is a fast and short-term response that occurs in the body in response to tissue injury, a twisted ankle, the common cold, bacteria, and virus infections. It lasts minutes to a day depending upon the impact of the injury. Acute inflammation is responsible to eliminate the cause of inflammation. It is one of the beneficial and necessary responses for tissue repair and recovery.

*Chronic inflammation* is one kind of persistent and long-term response that occurs in the body when our body's immune system fails to eliminate the cause of inflammation. Chronic inflammation lasts for an extended period, often months or even years, and is linked with various health conditions such as rheumatoid arthritis, diabetes, Alzheimer's, inflammatory bowel disease, atherosclerosis, and certain types of cancers. Symptoms of chronic inflammation include joint pain, skin issue, low energy, lower back pain, bloating, brain fog, poor digestion, and depression. Unhealthy eating habits, stressful work, lack of exercise, and smoking can be responsible for chronic inflammation.

# What is an Anti-Inflammatory Diet?

An anti-inflammatory diet is a dietary plan that focuses on eating foods that have been shown to have anti-inflammatory qualities, and minimizing or avoiding foods that can cause inflammation in the body. The goal is to reduce chronic inflammation, which is linked to different health problems and diseases. The diet promotes the intake of wholegrains, fruits, veggies, beans, nuts, and seeds. These foods are rich in vitamins, minerals, and fiber, and also come with antioxidant properties. This can help lower inflammation. An anti-inflammatory diet also includes Omega-3 foods like salmon, sardines, tuna, flaxseeds, walnuts, and chia seeds. This helps to boost the intake of Omega-3 fatty acids which come with anti-inflammatory properties.

An anti-inflammatory diet also reduces or eliminates the consumption of processed foods such as processed meat, sugary beverages, packaged snacks, fast food, etc. These foods promote inflammation in the body. An anti-inflammatory diet should be personalized to an individual's specific needs and health conditions. It is also important to consider other lifestyle factors such as enough sleep, regular physical exercise, and stress management as they may also affect inflammation levels in the body.

The anti-inflammatory diet helps you to cure medical conditions that involve inflammation such as rheumatoid arthritis, inflammatory bowel disease, cardiovascular, metabolic syndrome, and type 2 diabetes. It also helps you to maintain your body weight and prevent diseases. The purpose of an anti-inflammatory diet is to remove the inflammatory foods from your regular diet and introduce nutritious wholesome and nutrient-dense food into your diet. The anti-inflammatory diet helps you to cure chronic inflammation.

# Benefits of the Anti-Inflammatory Diet

The anti-inflammatory diet is a healthy eating habit that allows you to consume nutrient-dense foods that are a good source of vitamins, minerals, phytochemicals, Omega-3 fatty acids, micronutrients, and fibers. The diet is developed by a physician, and some of its benefits include:

- **Reduce chronic inflammation:** chronic inflammation has been linked with several health problems, including cardiovascular disease, obesity, diabetes, autoimmune diseases, and certain cancers. A diet that contains anti-inflammatory foods can aid in reducing the body's chronic inflammation, potentially reducing the risk and severity of certain illnesses. The anti-inflammatory diet is one of the healthiest methods of eating nutritious foods whether you are suffering from inflammation or not. The foods consumed during the anti-inflammatory diet are a rich source of essential vitamins, minerals, antioxidants, and fibers.

- **Healthy eating lifestyle:** the diet encourages you to consume nutrient-rich whole, minimally processed foods such as fruits, veggies, wholegrains, lean proteins, and healthy fats. These foods are nutrient-dense food and provide essential vitamins, minerals, phytochemicals, and antioxidants that support overall health. The diet is designed in such a way that you can get a balanced amount of carbohydrates, proteins, and fats. The diet inspires you to consume colorful fruits and vegetables such as dark green leafy vegetables, yellow fruits like oranges, tomatoes, berries, cruciferous veggies, and more.

- **Reduce the risk of heart disease:** adopting an anti-inflammatory diet has the potential to lower the chance of heart-related diseases. The anti-inflammatory diet is a good source of fibers and monounsaturated fats that help to increase the healthy HDL cholesterol level and reduce the unhealthy LDL cholesterol and triglyceride level. This balancing of cholesterol levels is excellent for heart health and also minimizes the risk of developing plaque in the arteries. The diet is a rich source of Omega-3 fatty acids. They can help reduce triglyceride levels, improve arterial function, lower blood pressure, and also reduce the risk of abnormal heart rhythms. The result leads to reduce the risk of cardiovascular disease, including strokes and heart attacks.

- **Reduce the risk of cancer:** some of the research and studies suggest that certain dietary patterns, including an anti-inflammatory diet, may be associated with a lower risk of certain types of cancers. The anti-inflammatory diet is rich in fruits, vegetables, wholegrains, and fish are also a good source of micronutrients, antioxidants, fibers, and phytonutrients, which helps to lower the risk of some cancers. In some cases, an anti-inflammatory diet reduces the risk of cancer by maintaining a healthy body weight.

- **Improved insulin sensitivity:** an anti-inflammatory diet can help control blood sugar levels and make insulin work better. By focusing on carbohydrates with a low glycemic index, cutting down on extra sugars, and putting more emphasis on fiber-rich foods, the diet can help balance blood sugar levels and possibly lower the risk of insulin resistance and type 2 diabetes.

- **Weight management:** an anti-inflammatory diet can help people who are trying to lose weight. The diet encourages you to consume whole, unprocessed foods that are low in added sugars, unhealthy fats, and refined carbohydrates. These foods tend to be more satiating and nutrient-dense, which can help keep you from feeling hungry and help you lose or maintain your body weight.

# Tips for Starting the Anti-Inflammatory Diet

1. **Learn diet basics:** what the anti-inflammatory diet is all about and how it works. Understand which foods are good for reducing inflammation and which ones make it worse. Familiarize yourself with the basic concepts and benefits of the diet.

2. **While consuming food, focus on whole, unprocessed foods:** base your meals on whole foods like fruits, veggies, lean meats, wholegrains, fatty fish, seeds, and nuts. Most of these foods are high in nutrients, vitamins, fiber, and come with antioxidant properties which can help reduce inflammation.

3. **Reduce intake of processed foods and added sugars:** processed foods contain unhealthy fats, refined carbs, and additives that can cause inflammation.

4. **Always choose lean protein:** if your goal is weight loss then you should eat lean protein. Lean sources of protein include fish, skinless poultry, lentils, and tofu. These protein sources are lower in saturated fat compared to red meats and can contribute to an overall anti-inflammatory eating pattern.

5. **Increase intake of fruits and vegetables:** pack your meal and snacks with colorful fruits and vegetables. These provide a wide range of vitamins, minerals, and phytonutrients that can help to fight against inflammation.

6. **Include healthy fats in your diet:** it is important to include healthy fats in your daily diet. These healthy fats include avocado, nuts, seeds, and olive oil which come with Omega-3 fatty acids and other compounds that have anti-inflammatory properties. Saturated and trans- fats, which are found in fried meals, processed foods, and high-fat meats, should be avoided during the diet.

7. **While purchasing packaged foods, always check the food label:** consider purchasing items with a minimal additive, preservative, and trans-fat content. Make sure there are no hidden sources of added sugars present, such as high-fructose corn syrup or other syrups.

8. **Maintain enough hydration:** consume a sufficient amount of water throughout the day to maintain enough hydration to support overall health. Reduce consumption of sugary drinks and switch to herbal tea, flavored water, or plain water instead.

# Key Anti-Inflammatory Ingredients and Pantry Staples

Anti-inflammatory food is one of the best sources of important vitamins, nutrients, minerals, and fibers and also has antioxidant properties. This helps to improve your immune system as well as brain functions and also helps to control your blood sugar level.

- **Fresh fruits:** Fruits are a rich source of vitamin C, minerals, nutrients, and antioxidants, which help to lower inflammation in your body. Use a lot of fruits with low glycemic index and a modest amount of fruits with high glycemic index, like apples, grapes, blackberries, papaya, plums, pineapple, avocado, watermelon, pomegranate, kiwi, and more.

- **Dark fresh leafy green vegetables:** vegetables are high in fiber and antioxidants, and they help to reduce inflammation. High-antioxidant vegetables include kale, spinach, Swiss chard, and romaine lettuce. Broccoli, bok choy, Brussels sprouts, and cauliflower are among the other veggies.

- **Wholegrains:** wholegrains such as millet, quinoa, and brown rice are the most effective gluten-free anti-inflammatory foods. You will get better outcomes if you consume wholegrains between three and five times every single day. When purchasing gluten-free whole cereals, you should always check the product's label for gluten-free certification.

- **Herbs and spices:** herbs and spices not only help to reduce inflammation but also enhance the flavor of your dish. Turmeric, black pepper, peppermint, cinnamon, thyme, ginger, cloves, rosemary, sage, and garlic are all herbs known as anti-inflammatory spices.

- **Choose healthy fats:** fats are an excellent source of energy. They provide 30 to 40 percent of the energy you need during the anti-inflammatory diet. It has been discovered that some kinds of good fats, such as the Omega-3 fatty acids that may be found in fatty fish, flaxseeds, chia seeds, hemp seeds, and walnuts, can reduce inflammation in the body. These fats have the potential to help reduce symptoms associated with chronic inflammatory disorders by lowering levels of inflammation in the body.

- **Consume seafood:** seafood is widely recognized as an excellent dietary choice due to its high protein content and plenty of Omega-3 fatty acids. Omega-3 fatty acids have been found to have positive effects on heart health, hormone regulation, and brain function. Seafood is known for its potential to reduce inflammation. Seafood includes a variety of fatty fish, such as salmon, albacore tuna, lake trout, sardines, and mackerel, as well as other options like shrimp, cod, and scallops.

- **Probiotics:** probiotics refer to beneficial bacteria, such as lactobacilli and bifid bacteria, which play a role in supporting the immune system. Probiotics have anti-inflammatory properties that aid in the treatment of constipation, diarrhea, and inflammatory diseases. Fermented dairy products, such as yogurt, kefir, and soy-based beverages help to increase the probiotic bacteria in our body.

# Chapter 2 - Breakfast Recipes

## The Place of Breakfast in the Anti-Inflammatory Diet

Breakfast is important in a diet that helps reduce inflammation. Breakfast is the first meal of the day and can influence your eating habits. Here is a short explanation of how breakfast fits into an anti-inflammatory diet. Having breakfast gives you the required energy to get the day started and fuels the activities you have planned. After going without food for the night, it helps your body recover by refueling your muscles and kick-starting your metabolism.

Eating a balanced breakfast helps you get important nutrients in your diet. When you eat foods that reduce inflammation, like fruits, vegetables, wholegrains, lean proteins, and healthy fats, you give your body important vitamins, minerals, antioxidants, and fiber. An anti-inflammatory breakfast is all about eating foods that can help decrease inflammation in the body. When you add ingredients like berries, leafy greens, turmeric, ginger, nuts and seeds, you bring in substances that can help reduce inflammation and improve your overall health.

Breakfast can also help to control your hunger for the rest of the day, making it less likely that you will eat unhealthy snacks or eat too much later. Foods that are high in protein, such as eggs, Greek yogurt, or plant-based proteins, can make you feel full and satisfied. It helps you be aware and focused on eating healthily, which makes it more likely that you will keep making choices that reduce inflammation throughout the day. If you choose to eat whole, unprocessed foods for breakfast, you can avoid or reduce the intake of ingredients that can cause inflammation in your body. These ingredients include refined grains, added sugars, unhealthy fats, and artificial additives that are often found in processed breakfast products.

Breakfast is an opportunity to rehydrate your body after sleep. Drinking water or herbal tea with your meal helps you to keep hydrated and also helps digestion. Don't forget, breakfast is an important part of a diet that fights inflammation. Choosing healthy anti-inflammatory ingredients for your morning meal can help you live a healthier life.

# 1 - Berry Spinach Smoothie

**Preparation time: 5 minutes**

**Cooking time: 5 minutes**

**Serves: 2**

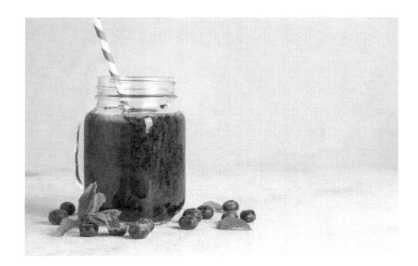

## Ingredients:

- 1 cup fresh spinach
- 4 tbsp rolled oats
- 1 banana
- 2 cups mixed berries
- 1 cup unsweetened almond milk

## Directions:

- Add spinach and remaining ingredients into the blender and blend until smooth.

- Serve immediately and enjoy.

## Nutritional value (amount per serving):

- Calories 195
- Fat 3.2g
- Carbohydrates 39g
- Sugar 17.4g
- Protein 3.9g
- Cholesterol 0mg

# 2 - Overnight Chia Pudding

**Preparation time: 10 minutes**

**Cooking time: 5 minutes**

**Serves: 4**

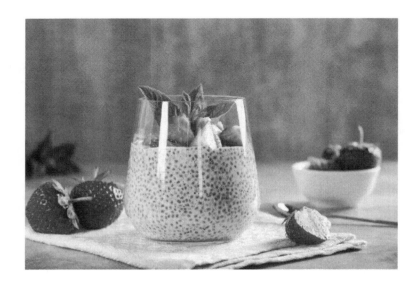

## Ingredients:

- ¼ cup chia seeds
- 2 ½ tsp maple syrup
- 1 tsp vanilla extract
- ½ cup Greek yogurt
- 1 cup unsweetened almond milk

## Directions:

- In a bowl, add chia seeds, yogurt, and almond milk and mix until well blended.
- Add maple syrup and vanilla extract and whisk well.
- Cover and place in the fridge overnight.
- Top with fresh berries and serve.

## Nutritional value (amount per serving):

- Calories 51
- Fat 1.9g
- Carbohydrates 5.2g
- Sugar 3.6g
- Protein 3.1g
- Cholesterol 1mg

# 3 - Vegetable Omelet

**Preparation time: 10 minutes**

**Cooking time: 10 minutes**

**Serves: 2**

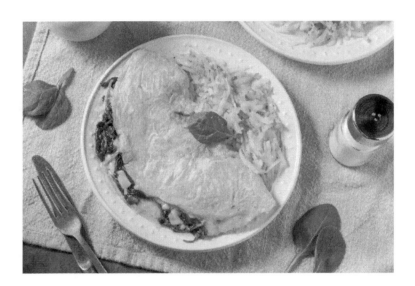

## Ingredients:

- 4 eggs
- 1 tbsp olive oil
- ¼ cup Parmesan cheese, shredded
- ¼ cup leek, sliced
- ½ cup cherry tomatoes, cut in half
- ½ cup baby spinach
- 2 tbsp whipping cream
- 1/8 tsp cayenne pepper

- Pepper
- Salt

**Directions:**

- Heat olive oil in a pan over medium-low heat.
- In a bowl, whisk eggs with whipping cream, pepper, and salt.
- Add egg mixture to the pan and cook over low heat.
- Once the omelet starts to set then add leek, spinach, tomatoes, and Parmesan cheese. Season with cayenne pepper, pepper, and salt.
- Once the omelet is completely set then gently fold the omelet in half and cook over low heat until cheese melts.
- Cut in half and serve.

**Nutritional value (amount per serving):**

- Calories 258
- Fat 21.3g
- Carbohydrates 4.3g
- Sugar 2.4g
- Protein 2g
- Cholesterol 347mg

# 4 - Quinoa Breakfast Bowl

**Preparation time: 10 minutes**

**Cooking time: 15 minutes**

**Serves: 1**

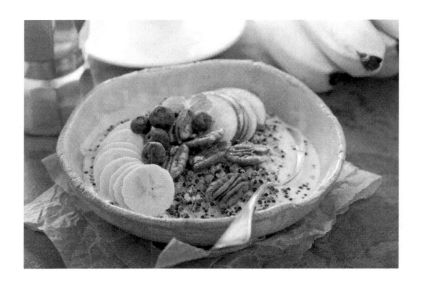

## Ingredients:

- ¼ cup quinoa, rinsed
- 1 tbsp pumpkin seeds
- 1 tbsp slivered almonds
- 1 tbsp walnuts, chopped
- ¼ cup blueberries
- 1/8 tsp vanilla extract
- 1/8 tsp cinnamon
- 1 tbsp maple syrup

- ¼ cup unsweetened almond milk
- ½ banana, mashed
- ½ banana, sliced
- 2 tbsp dried cranberries
- ¾ cup water

## Directions:

- Add ½ cup of water in a saucepan and bring to boil. Add quinoa. Turn heat to low, cover and simmer for 12-15 minutes or until liquid is absorbed.
- Once quinoa is cooked then remove from heat and fluff with a fork.
- Add mashed banana, vanilla, cinnamon, maple syrup, and almond milk to the cooked quinoa and mix well.
- Transfer quinoa mixture to the serving bowl and top with banana slices, cranberries, pumpkin seeds, almonds, walnuts, and blueberries.
- Serve and enjoy.

## Nutritional value (amount per serving):

- Calories 121
- Fat 3.9g
- Carbohydrates 19.6g
- Sugar 7.7g
- Protein 3.3g
- Cholesterol 0mg

# 5 - Golden Turmeric Latte

**Preparation time: 10 minutes**

**Cooking time: 5 minutes**

**Serves: 2**

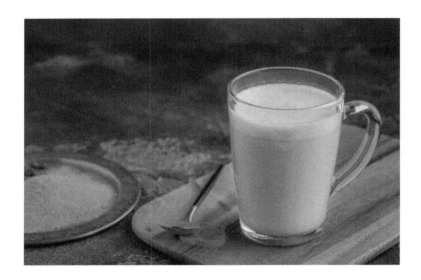

## Ingredients:

- 2 cups unsweetened almond milk
- ½ tsp vanilla extract
- Pinch of cayenne
- Pinch of black pepper
- ¼ tsp ginger powder
- ½ tsp cinnamon
- ½ tsp turmeric
- 1 tbsp maple syrup

## Directions:

- Add all ingredients into the small pot, whisk well and heat over medium-high heat until just comes to a boil.
- Pour into the two serving cups.
- Serve immediately and enjoy.

## Nutritional value (amount per serving):

- Calories 74
- Fat 3.6g
- Carbohydrates 9.9g
- Sugar 6.1g
- Protein 1.1g
- Cholesterol 0mg

# 6 - Banana Walnut Muffins

**Preparation time: 10 minutes**

**Cooking time: 20 minutes**

**Serves: 9**

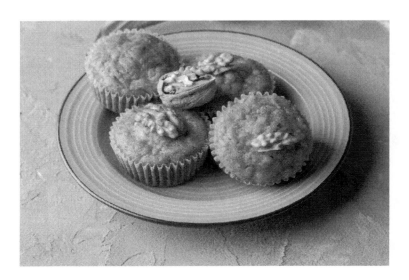

## Ingredients:

- 1 cup mashed banana
- 1 tsp apple cider vinegar
- 1 tsp vanilla
- 2 eggs
- 1/3 cup coconut oil, melted
- ¼ cup walnuts, chopped
- ¼ tsp cinnamon
- 1 tsp baking soda
- 1 tbsp ground flaxseeds

- ½ cup cassava flour
- ¼ tsp sea salt

## Directions:

- Preheat the oven to 350F.
- Line muffin pan with muffin liners and set aside.
- In a mixing bowl, add mashed bananas, vinegar, vanilla, eggs, and oil and whisk until well combined.
- Add cassava flour, cinnamon, baking soda, ground flaxseeds, and salt and stir until combined.
- Add chopped walnuts and fold well.
- Spoon batter into each muffin liner and bake in preheated oven for 20 minutes.
- Serve and enjoy.

## Nutritional value (amount per serving):

- Calories 144
- Fat 11.5g
- Carbohydrates 9g
- Sugar 2.2g
- Protein 2.5g
- Cholesterol 36mg

# 7 - Avocado Toast with Smoked Salmon

**Preparation time: 10 minutes**

**Cooking time: 10 minutes**

**Serves: 2**

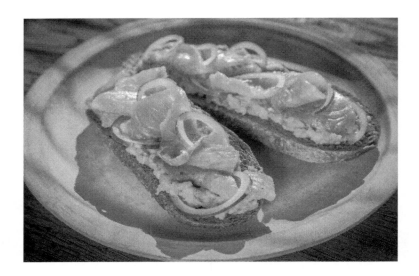

## Ingredients:

- 2 large bread slices
- ¼ cup onion, cut into thin slices
- 10 capers
- 2oz smoked salmon, thinly sliced
- ½ lemon juice
- 1 avocado; scoop out the flesh
- Pepper
- Salt

## Directions:

- In a small bowl, add avocado flesh and mash using a fork. Add lemon juice, pepper, and salt and mix well.
- Toast bread slices. Spread avocado mixture on toasted bread slices and top with capers.
- Top avocado with a salmon slice and onion slices.
- Serve immediately and enjoy.

## Nutritional value (amount per serving):

- Calories 302
- Fat 21.3g
- Carbohydrates 21.9g
- Sugar 2g
- Protein 10.4g
- Cholesterol 7mg

# 8 - Blueberry Oatmeal Breakfast Bars

**Preparation time: 10 minutes**

**Cooking time: 30 minutes**

**Serves: 12**

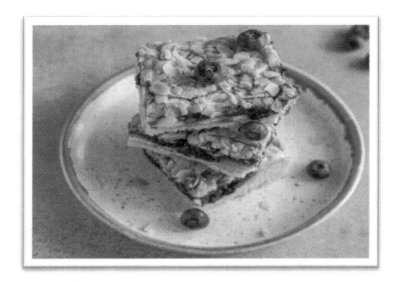

## Ingredients:

- 2 eggs
- 2 cups quick-rolled oats
- 1 cup blueberries
- 1 tsp cinnamon
- 1 tsp baking powder
- 1 tsp vanilla extract
- ¼ cup coconut oil, melted
- ½ cup coconut sugar

- 1 cup unsweetened almond milk
- 1 cup oat flour
- ¼ tsp salt

## Directions:

- Line an 11x7-inch baking dish with parchment paper and set aside.
- Preheat the oven to 350F.
- In a mixing bowl, whisk together eggs, coconut oil, vanilla, milk, and coconut sugar.
- Add oats, cinnamon, baking powder, oat flour, and salt and mix until well combined.
- Add blueberries and fold well.
- Pour batter into the prepared baking dish and bake in preheated oven for 30-35 minutes. Remove the baking dish from oven and allow to cool completely.
- Remove bars from the baking dish and cut into pieces.
- Serve and enjoy.

## Nutritional value (amount per serving):

- Calories 159
- Fat 7.3g
- Carbohydrates 19.8g
- Sugar 1.5g
- Protein 4.3g
- Cholesterol 27mg

# 9 - Sweet Potato & Kale Breakfast Skillet

**Preparation time: 10 minutes**

**Cooking time: 10 minutes**

**Serves: 4**

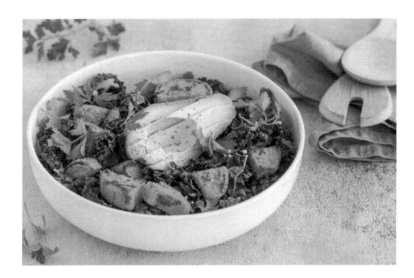

## Ingredients:

- 1 sweet potato, cut into ¼-inch cubes
- 8oz mushrooms, sliced
- 10 kale stalks, stems removed & chopped
- 1 tbsp garlic, minced
- 1 onion, chopped
- 1 tbsp olive oil
- Pepper

- Salt

## Directions:

- Heat olive oil in a large skillet over medium heat.
- Add onion to the skillet and sauté for 3 minutes. Add garlic and sauté for minute.
- Add sweet potatoes, pepper, and salt and cook for 5 minutes.
- Add chopped kale and mushrooms and cook until mushrooms soften.
- Serve and enjoy.

## Nutritional value (amount per serving):

- Calories 165
- Fat 3.8g
- Carbohydrates 28.5g
- Sugar 4g
- Protein 7.8g
- Cholesterol 0mg

# 10 - Healthy Scrambled Eggs

**Preparation time: 5 minutes**

**Cooking time: 20 minutes**

**Serves: 6**

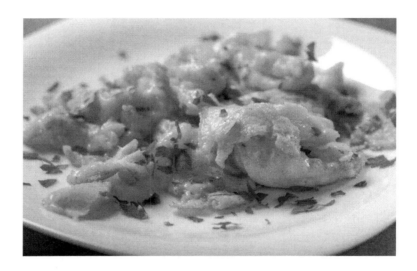

## Ingredients:

- 10 eggs
- 1 tsp turmeric powder
- ½ cup unsweetened almond milk
- ¼ tsp ground cumin
- 2 tbsp fresh cilantro, chopped
- Pepper
- Salt

## Directions:

- Preheat the oven to 350F.
- In a bowl, whisk eggs with turmeric, cumin, milk, pepper, and salt.
- Pour egg mixture into the greased casserole dish and place in preheated oven for 10-12 minutes or until eggs have started to set.
- Remove casserole dish from oven and using spatula stir eggs.
- Return casserole dish to the oven for 8-10 minutes or until eggs are set.
- Remove from oven and stir again with spatula.
- Garnish with cilantro and serve.

## Nutritional value (amount per serving):

- Calories 110
- Fat 7.6g
- Carbohydrates 1g
- Sugar 0.6g
- Protein 9.4g
- Cholesterol 273mg

# 11 - Almond Butter Banana Wrap

**Preparation time: 10 minutes**

**Cooking time: 5 minutes**

**Serves: 1**

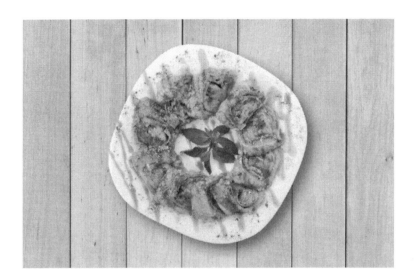

**Ingredients:**

- 1 low-carb wheat wrap
- 1 small banana, sliced
- 1 tbsp almond butter

**Directions:**

- Lay the wheat wrap out flat and spread almond butter over the top.

- Arrange banana slices on the almond butter and then roll up the wrap.
- Cut into slices and serve.

## Nutritional value (amount per serving):

- Calories 263
- Fat 12.8g
- Carbohydrates 37.1g
- Sugar 14.1g
- Protein 12.5g
- Cholesterol 0mg

# 12 - Veggie Breakfast Burrito

**Preparation time: 10 minutes**

**Cooking time: 10 minutes**

**Serves: 2**

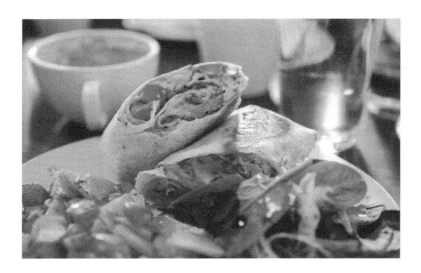

## Ingredients:

- 2 tortillas
- ¼ cup cilantro, chopped
- ¼ cup Parmesan cheese, grated
- 4 eggs, lightly beaten
- 4 tbsp black beans, cooked
- 1 small tomato, chopped
- ¼ red bell pepper, chopped
- 1 tbsp olive oil
- ½ small onion, chopped

- Pepper
- Salt

## Directions:

- Heat olive oil in a pan over medium heat.
- Add onion to the pan and sauté until softened.
- Add bell pepper and tomato and cook for 2-3 minutes. Add beans and mix well.
- Add eggs and stir constantly until eggs are completely cooked. Season with pepper and salt. Remove pan from heat.
- Meanwhile warm the tortillas in a frying pan.
- Add cilantro and grated cheese to the egg mixture and mix well.
- Fill the tortillas with egg and vegetable mixture and serve immediately.

## Nutritional value (amount per serving):

- Calories 377
- Fat 19.3g
- Carbohydrates 31.5g
- Sugar 4.1g
- Protein 22.1g
- Cholesterol 335mg

# 13 - Buckwheat Pancakes with Fresh Berries

**Preparation time: 10 minutes**

**Cooking time: 10 minutes**

**Serves: 6**

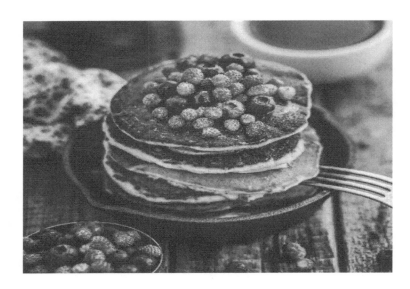

## Ingredients:

- 1 egg
- 2 tsp baking powder
- 1 tbsp flaxmeal
- 1 cup buckwheat flour
- ¼ cup unsweetened almond milk
- 1/3 cup Greek yogurt
- 2 medium bananas, mashed

- Pinch of cinnamon
- Salt

## Directions:

- In a mixing bowl, whisk together egg, mashed bananas, milk, and yogurt until well combined.
- In a separate bowl, mix together flour, baking powder, flaxmeal, cinnamon, and salt.
- Add flour mixture into the egg mixture and mix until just combined.
- Spray a large pan with cooking spray and heat over medium heat.
- Spoon a ¼ cup batter onto a hot pan and cook for 2-3 minutes, turn the pancake and cook for 1 minute. Make remaining batter pancakes.
- Serve pancakes with berries.

## Nutritional value (amount per serving):

- Calories 129
- Fat 2.3g
- Carbohydrates 24.8g
- Sugar 5.8g
- Protein 5.3g
- Cholesterol 28mg

# 14 - Mushroom & Spinach Egg Muffins

**Preparation time: 10 minutes**

**Cooking time: 30 minutes**

**Serves: 12**

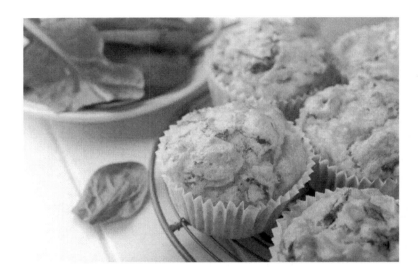

## Ingredients:

- 12 eggs
- 2 cups Asiago cheese, shredded
- ¼ cup unsweetened almond milk
- 1 tbsp olive oil
- 1 cup spinach, chopped
- 6 oz mushrooms, sliced
- Pepper
- Salt

## Directions:

- Spray muffin pan with cooking spray and set aside.
- Preheat the oven to 350F.
- Heat olive oil in a pan over medium heat.
- Add mushrooms and sauté until softened. Add spinach and cook until it's wilted, about 2-3 minutes.
- Divide mushroom spinach mixture among each muffin cup.
- In a bowl, whisk together eggs, milk, pepper, and salt. Stir in shredded cheese.
- Pour egg mixture evenly into each muffin cup.
- Bake in preheated oven for 25 minutes.
- Serve and enjoy.

## Nutritional value (amount per serving):

- Calories 78
- Fat 5.7g
- Carbohydrates 1g
- Sugar 0.6g
- Protein 6.1g
- Cholesterol 164mg

# 15 - Quinoa Banana Bread

**Preparation time: 10 minutes**

**Cooking time: 30 minutes**

**Serves: 8**

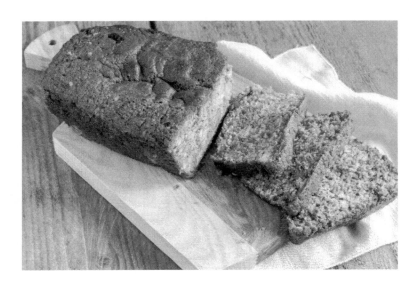

## Ingredients:

- 2 eggs
- 1 cup quinoa flour
- 3 bananas, mashed
- 1 tsp vanilla extract
- 2 tbsp honey
- 1 tsp baking powder
- 1 tsp baking soda
- ¼ cup flaxseed meal

- ¼ tsp salt

## Directions:

- Preheat the oven to 350F.
- Spray a 9x5-inch loaf pan with cooking spray and set aside.
- In a mixing bowl, whisk together eggs, mashed bananas, vanilla, and honey until well combined.
- In a separate bowl, mix together quinoa flour, baking powder, baking soda, and flaxseed meal.
- Add the quinoa flour mixture to the egg mixture and mix until well combined.
- Pour batter into the prepared loaf pan and bake in preheated oven for 30 minutes until done.
- Remove the loaf pan from oven and allow to cool completely.
- Slice and serve.

## Nutritional value (amount per serving):

- Calories 158
- Fat 3.3g
- Carbohydrates 27.4g
- Sugar 10.4g
- Protein 4.5g
- Cholesterol 41mg

# Chapter 3 - Appetizer and Snack Recipes

## The Place of Appetizers and Snacks in the Anti-Inflammatory Diet

Appetizers and snacks are essential parts of a diet that helps to reduce the inflammation in the body and can also have a positive impact on overall general health and well-being.

**Appetizers:** Appetizers are nothing but small dishes served before a meal to make you hungry. An anti-inflammatory diet allows you to eat nutrient-rich foods that are good for you and can help reduce inflammation. Appetizers can be made with ingredients like fresh vegetables, fruits, lean proteins, and healthy fats. These healthy foods are a rich source of vitamins, minerals, antioxidants, and fiber. They help to keep you healthy and fight against inflammation. Starting your main meal with a healthy appetizer can make you satisfied and stop you from eating too much unhealthy food.

**Snacks:** Snacks are used as energy boosters in-between meals when following an anti-inflammatory diet. They give sustained energy throughout the day and aid in keeping blood sugar levels in control. Healthy snacks can reduce hunger and stop overeating during meals. Protein, healthy fats, and fiber-rich snacks can help you feel satiated and keep you feeling full between meals. Snacks give you a chance to add more fruits, vegetables, wholegrains, and other ingredients that help reduce inflammation in your diet. This helps make sure that are meeting your nutritional needs and supporting overall health. If you have healthy snacks easily accessible, you won't need to depend on processed or unhealthy food choices. Choose natural foods such as fresh fruits, raw nuts, yogurt, or homemade snacks to minimize the consumption of inflammatory ingredients. It's important to watch how much you eat snacks. Pre-portioning snacks or choosing single-serving options can help you avoid eating too many calories and also helps to control your weight.

In an anti-inflammatory diet, it's important to choose appetizers and snacks that use whole, unprocessed foods. Try to avoid ingredients like refined grains, added sugars, unhealthy fats, and artificial additives, as they can cause inflammation. If you choose wisely and pick foods that are good for you, it can help your health and lower inflammation in your body.

# 1 - Guacamole with Veggie Sticks

**Preparation time: 10 minutes**

**Cooking time: 5 minutes**

**Serves: 3**

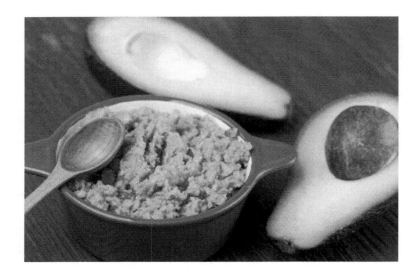

### Ingredients:

- 2 large avocados; scoop out the flesh
- 2 garlic cloves, minced
- ¼ cup fresh cilantro, chopped
- 1 tbsp lime juice
- Salt

### Directions:

- Add avocado flesh into the bowl and mash using a fork.

- Add remaining ingredients and mix until well combined.
- Serve guacamole with vegetable sticks.

**Nutritional value (amount per serving):**

- Calories 280
- Fat 26.2g
- Carbohydrates 13.5g
- Sugar 1g
- Protein 2.8g
- Cholesterol 0mg

# 2 - Hummus with Wholegrain Crackers

**Preparation time: 10 minutes**

**Cooking time: 5 minutes**

**Serves: 4**

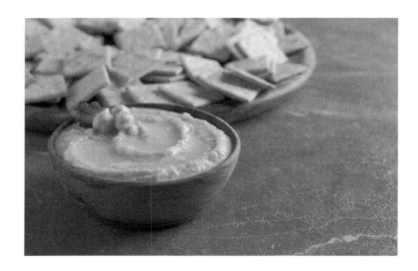

## Ingredients:

- 2½ cups cooked chickpeas
- 1/3 cup water
- 2 garlic cloves
- Juice of half a lemon
- 1 tbsp soy sauce, low-sodium
- 2 tbsp sesame Tahini
- Salt

## Directions:

- Add chickpeas and remaining ingredients into the food processor and process until smooth.
- Serve hummus with wholewheat crackers or roasted veggies.

## Nutritional value (amount per serving):

- Calories 681
- Fat 16.8g
- Carbohydrates 103.7g
- Sugar 18.1g
- Protein 35g
- Cholesterol 0mg

# 3 - Cucumber Avocado Roll-Ups

**Preparation time: 10 minutes**

**Cooking time: 10 minutes**

**Serves: 12**

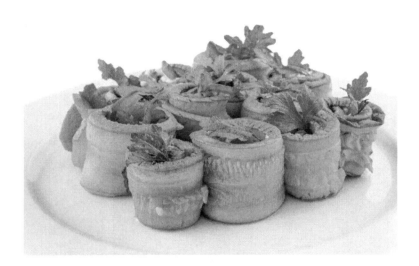

## Ingredients:

- 1 English cucumber, cut into long, thin strips
- 1 avocado; scoop out the flesh
- 1 garlic clove
- 2 tsp lime juice
- ¼ cup fresh basil
- Pepper
- Salt

## Directions:

- Add avocado flesh, garlic, lime juice, basil, pepper, and salt into the blender and blend until smooth.
- Take one cucumber strip and spread a thin layer of avocado mixture along the length of the cucumber and roll it up. Make remaining cucumber rolls.
- Serve and enjoy.

## Nutritional value (amount per serving):

- Calories 24
- Fat 2g
- Carbohydrates 1.9g
- Sugar 0.4g
- Protein 0.3g
- Cholesterol 0mg

# 4 – Roasted Chickpeas with Turmeric

**Preparation time: 10 minutes**

**Cooking time: 40 minutes**

**Serves: 4**

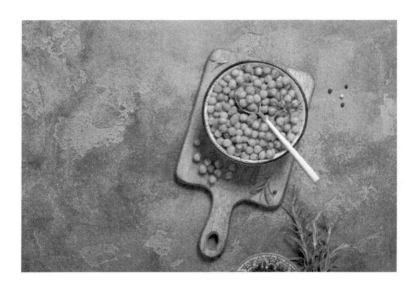

## Ingredients:

- 14.5oz can chickpeas, drained & rinsed
- 2 tsp olive oil
- ½ tsp paprika
- 1 tsp turmeric
- ¼ tsp black pepper
- 1 tsp salt

## Directions:

- In a bowl, toss chickpeas with olive oil, paprika, turmeric, pepper, and salt until well coated.
- Spread chickpeas onto a parchment-lined baking sheet.
- Roast at 350F for 20 minutes. Stir chickpeas and bake for 20 minutes more.
- Remove chickpeas from oven and allow to cool completely.
- Serve and enjoy.

## Nutritional value (amount per serving):

- Calories 145
- Fat 3.6g
- Carbohydrates 23.8g
- Sugar 0.1g
- Protein 5.2g
- Cholesterol 0mg

# 5 – Smoked Salmon Cucumber Bites

**Preparation time: 10 minutes**

**Cooking time: 5 minutes**

**Serves: 30**

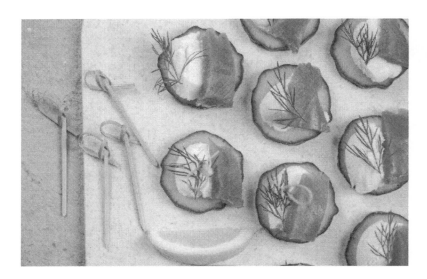

## Ingredients:

- 1 large English cucumber, peeled & cut into 1/3-inch slices
- 7oz smoked salmon, cut into pieces
- 1 tsp lemon juice
- 1 tbsp dill, chopped
- 1 tbsp unsweetened almond milk
- 6oz cream cheese
- Pepper
- Salt

## Directions:

- In a small bowl, mix together cream cheese, lemon juice, dill, milk, pepper, and salt.
- Spread cream cheese mixture over each cucumber slice, then top with smoked salmon pieces.
- Serve and enjoy.

## Nutritional value (amount per serving):

- Calories 28
- Fat 2.3g
- Carbohydrates 0.3g
- Sugar 0g
- Protein 1.7g
- Cholesterol 0mg

# 6 – Turmeric Cashew Coconut Energy Bites

**Preparation time: 10 minutes**

**Cooking time: 10 minutes**

**Serves: 12**

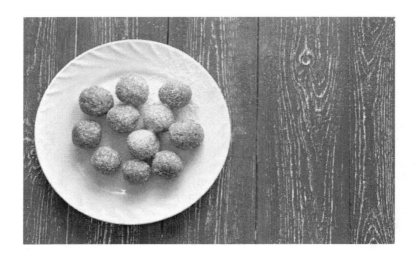

## Ingredients:

- 1½ cups cashews
- ¼ tsp turmeric
- 1 cup shredded coconut
- 1 tbsp coconut oil, melted
- 2 tbsp honey
- ¼ cup apple cider vinegar
- Juice from 2 lemons
- ½ grated zest of one lemon

## Directions:

- Add cashews and remaining ingredients into the food processor and process until sticky dough forms.
- Make equal-shaped balls from mixture and place onto a parchment-lined baking sheet.
- Store in refrigerator for up to one week.
- Serve and enjoy.

## Nutritional value (amount per serving):

- Calories 144
- Fat 11.3g
- Carbohydrates 9.5g
- Sugar 4g
- Protein 2.9g
- Cholesterol 0mg

# 7 - Spiced Roasted Nuts

**Preparation time: 10 minutes**

**Cooking time: 20 minutes**

**Serves: 16**

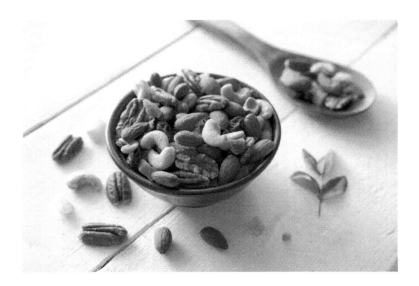

## Ingredients:

- 1 cup cashews
- 1 cup almonds
- 1 cup walnuts
- 1 cup pecans
- 2 tbsp olive oil
- ½ tsp chili powder
- ½ tsp smoked paprika
- 1 tsp dried dill

- 1 tsp onion powder
- 1 tsp garlic powder
- ½ tsp kosher salt

## Directions:

- Preheat the oven to 325F.
- Add nuts and remaining ingredients into the mixing bowl and toss until well coated.
- Spread nuts onto a parchment-lined baking sheet and roast in preheated oven for 20 minutes. Stir halfway through.
- Remove from oven and allow to cool completely.
- Serve and enjoy.

## Nutritional value (amount per serving):

- Calories 155
- Fat 14g
- Carbohydrates 5.3g
- Sugar 0.9g
- Protein 4.6g
- Cholesterol 0mg

# 8 - Greek Yogurt Dip with Fresh Vegetables

**Preparation time: 5 minutes**

**Cooking time: 5 minutes**

**Serves: 6**

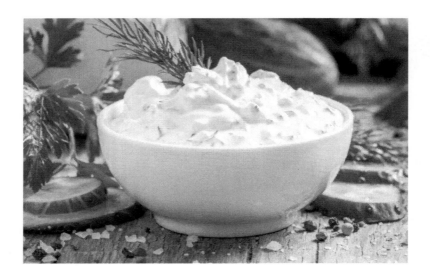

## Ingredients:

- 1½ cups plain Greek yogurt
- 2 tbsp unsweetened almond milk
- 1 tsp garlic powder
- 1 tsp onion powder
- 1 tsp dried dill
- 1 tsp Italian seasoning
- ¼ tsp pepper

- ½ tsp garlic salt

## Directions:

- In a small bowl, whisk together yogurt, milk, garlic powder, onion powder, dill, Italian seasoning, pepper, and garlic salt until smooth and creamy.
- Serve with fresh veggies.

## Nutritional value (amount per serving):

- Calories 28
- Fat 0.3g
- Carbohydrates 2.6g
- Sugar 1.9g
- Protein 4g
- Cholesterol 2mg

# 9 - Sweet Potato Fries with Turmeric Dip

**Preparation time: 10 minutes**

**Cooking time: 40 minutes**

**Serves: 4**

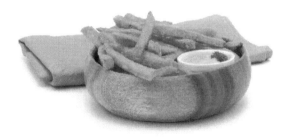

## Ingredients:

- 4 medium sweet potatoes, thinly sliced
- Pinch of cayenne
- 2 tbsp olive oil
- Pepper
- Salt
- For the turmeric dip:
- 2 tbsp Tahini

- 1 tbsp maple syrup
- ½ tsp turmeric
- 2 tbsp hot water
- ¼ tsp pepper
- ¼ tsp sea salt

## Directions:

- Preheat the oven to 425F.
- In a large bowl, toss sweet potato slices with cayenne, olive oil, pepper, and salt until well coated.
- Arrange sweet potato slices onto a parchment-lined baking sheet and bake in preheated oven for 40 minutes. Flip halfway through.
- For the dip: in a small bowl, whisk together Tahini, maple syrup, turmeric, hot water, pepper, and salt until smooth.
- Serve sweet potato fries with turmeric dip.

## Nutritional value (amount per serving):

- Calories 296
- Fat 11.3g
- Carbohydrates 47.1g
- Sugar 3.8g
- Protein 3.6g
- Cholesterol 0mg

# 10 - Caprese Skewers with Balsamic Glaze

**Preparation time: 10 minutes**

**Cooking time: 5 minutes**

**Serves: 20 skewers**

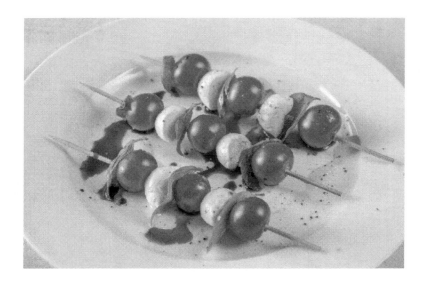

## Ingredients:

- 6oz mozzarella balls
- 2 tbsp balsamic reduction
- 1 cup fresh basil leaves
- 4 cups cherry tomatoes
- 2 tbsp olive oil
- ½ tsp Italian seasoning
- Pepper

- Salt

## Directions:

- In a mixing bowl, toss mozzarella balls with Italian seasoning and olive oil.
- Thread cherry tomatoes, basil, and mozzarella balls onto a wooden skewer. Make remaining skewers.
- Arrange skewers onto a serving plate and season with pepper and salt. Drizzle with balsamic reduction.
- Serve and enjoy.

## Nutritional value (amount per serving):

- Calories 49
- Fat 3.3g
- Carbohydrates 3.1g
- Sugar 2.3g
- Protein 2.4g
- Cholesterol 6mg

## 11 - Zucchini Pizza Bites

**Preparation time: 10 minutes**

**Cooking time: 5 minutes**

**Serves: 6**

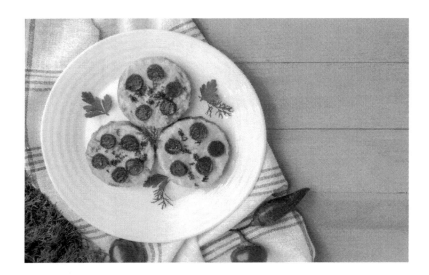

### Ingredients:

- 2 large zucchini, cut into ¼-inch thick slices
- ¼ cup Parmesan cheese, grated
- 2 cups mozzarella cheese, shredded
- 1 tsp oregano
- ½ cup pizza sauce, low-carb
- Pizza toppings as desired

### Directions:

- Preheat the oven to 450F.

- Top each zucchini slice with pizza sauce, cheese, oregano, and your favorite pizza toppings.
- Arrange zucchini slices onto a parchment-lined baking sheet and bake in preheated oven for 5 minutes.

**Nutritional value (amount per serving):**

- Calories 88
- Fat 2.1g
- Carbohydrates 7.1g
- Sugar 2.5g
- Protein 7g
- Cholesterol 8mg

# 12 - Almond Butter Energy Balls

**Preparation time: 10 minutes**

**Cooking time: 5 minutes**

**Serves: 16**

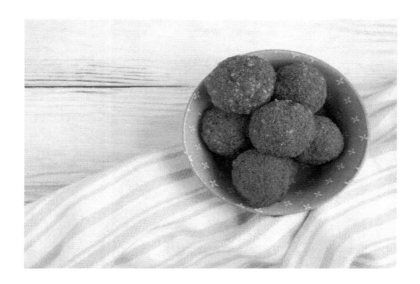

## Ingredients:

- ½ cup almond butter
- ½ tsp cinnamon
- 1 tsp vanilla extract
- 1 tbsp maple syrup
- ½ cup rolled oats
- 10 Medjool dates, pitted
- 1 cup almonds
- ¼ tsp salt

## Directions:

- Add almond butter and remaining ingredients into the food processor and process until sticky dough forms.
- Roll into equally-shaped balls and serve.

## Nutritional value (amount per serving):

- Calories 139
- Fat 3.4g
- Carbohydrates 26.5g
- Sugar 19.2g
- Protein 2.3g
- Cholesterol 42mg

# 13 - Beetroot & Goat Cheese Crostini

**Preparation time: 10 minutes**

**Cooking time: 1 hour 5 minutes**

**Serves: 4**

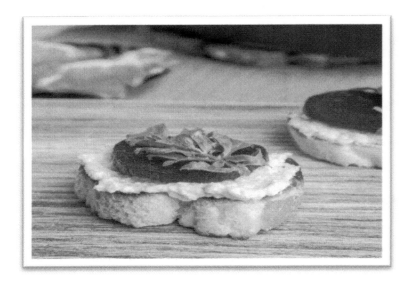

## Ingredients:

- 10 wholewheat baguette slices, toasted
- 4oz goat cheese, softened
- 1 large beet, scrubbed
- 1 tbsp vinegar
- 2 tbsp olive oil
- 2 tbsp parsley, chopped
- 1 garlic clove, minced
- ½ tsp salt

## Directions:

- Preheat the oven to 400F.
- Wrap beetroot in foil and bake in preheated oven for 50-60 minutes. Remove from oven and allow to cool completely.
- Once the beet is cool then remove the peel and dice into small pieces.
- In a bowl, mix together beets, vinegar, olive oil, parsley, garlic, and salt.
- Spread cheese on baguette slices then spoon beet mixture on top of each baguette slice.
- Serve and enjoy.

## Nutritional value (amount per serving):

- Calories 431
- Fat 18.6g
- Carbohydrates 48.3g
- Sugar 4.4g
- Protein 18.5g
- Cholesterol 30mg

# 14 - Kale Chips with Garlic & Sea Salt

**Preparation time: 5 minutes**

**Cooking time: 15 minutes**

**Serves: 4**

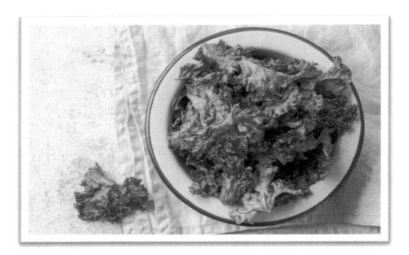

## Ingredients:

- 4 cups kale leaves, cut into small pieces
- 1/8 tsp smoked paprika
- 1/8 tsp garlic powder
- 2 tbsp olive oil
- Pinch of sea salt

## Directions:

- Preheat the oven to 350F.

- In a mixing bowl, add kale then pour olive oil over kale and mix until kale is well coated.
- Sprinkle paprika, garlic powder, and salt over the kale then spread the kale onto a baking sheet.
- Bake in preheated oven for 15 minutes. Remove from oven and allow to cool completely.
- Serve and enjoy.

**Nutritional value (amount per serving):**

- Calories 94
- Fat 7g
- Carbohydrates 7.1g
- Sugar 0g
- Protein 2g
- Cholesterol 0mg

# 15 - Cinnamon Apple Chips

**Preparation time: 10 minutes**

**Cooking time: 14 minutes**

**Serves: 2**

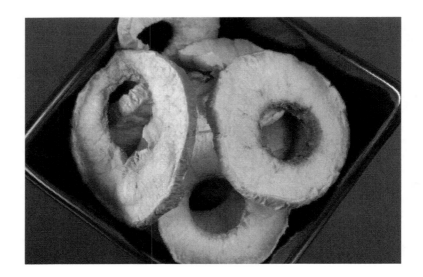

## Ingredients:

- 2 apples, cut into 1/8-inch thick slices
- 1 tsp ground cinnamon

## Directions:

- Arrange the apple slices onto a large baking sheet and sprinkle the cinnamon on top.
- Working in batches, add apple slices into the air-fryer basket and cook at 300F for 14 minutes. Flip halfway through.

- Remove apple chips from the air-fryer and allow to cool completely.
- Serve and enjoy.

## Nutritional value (amount per serving):

- Calories 119
- Fat 0.4g
- Carbohydrates 31.7g
- Sugar 23.2g
- Protein 0.7g
- Cholesterol 0mg

# Chapter 4 - Salad Recipes

## The Place of Salads in the Anti-Inflammatory Diet

Salads are good for an anti-inflammatory diet because they have many health benefits. They contain lots of fresh veggies that are full of important vitamins, minerals, and antioxidants. These nutrients help your immune system, reduce inflammation, and make you healthier. Salads usually have lots of fiber from veggies. This helps with digestion, makes you feel full, and keeps your blood sugar levels steady. Fiber helps keep your gut healthy, which can help reduce inflammation. Salads made with ingredients like cucumbers, tomatoes, and lettuce contain a lot of water. Eating a salad can help you stay hydrated and support your overall health.

Salads contain leafy greens and colorful vegetables that are high in antioxidants. These antioxidants help to defend your body against oxidative stress as well as inflammation-related damage. Healthy fats, such as Omega-3 fatty acids and monounsaturated fats, can be added to salads by using items like avocado, almonds, or seeds. These fats are beneficial for heart health and contain anti-inflammatory properties. Consuming salad at the beginning of a meal can help limit portion sizes and calorie intake. Salads are high in fiber content that makes you feel satisfied and helps you prevent overeating.

In an anti-inflammatory diet, salads are best when made with fresh, nutrient-dense foods and without processed dressings, croutons, or excessive cheese. Salads are healthy and delicious, and help to lower inflammation.

# 1 - Mixed Greens Salad with Berries & Walnuts

**Preparation time: 10 minutes**

**Cooking time: 10 minutes**

**Serves: 4**

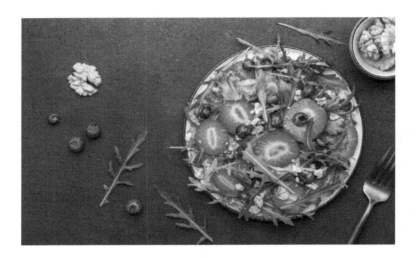

## Ingredients:

- 5oz mixed salad greens
- 1/3 cup walnuts, toasted
- 1 avocado, diced
- 1 cup blueberries
- 1 cup raspberries
- 1 cup strawberries, quartered
- For the dressing:
- ¼ cup avocado oil

- 1/8 tsp garlic powder
- 2 tbsp honey
- 1 tbsp lemon juice
- 2 tbsp red wine vinegar
- ¼ tsp pepper
- ½ tsp salt

## Directions:

- In a small bowl, whisk together all dressing ingredients until well combined. Set aside.
- In a large bowl, mix together salad greens, walnuts, avocado, blueberries, raspberries, and strawberries.
- Pour dressing over salad and toss well.
- Serve and enjoy.

## Nutritional value (amount per serving):

- Calories 275
- Fat 18.2g
- Carbohydrates 27.9g
- Sugar 15.9g
- Protein 5.1g
- Cholesterol 0mg

# 2 - Kale & Quinoa Salad with Lemon Tahini Dressing

**Preparation time: 10 minutes**

**Cooking time: 5 minutes**

**Serves: 1**

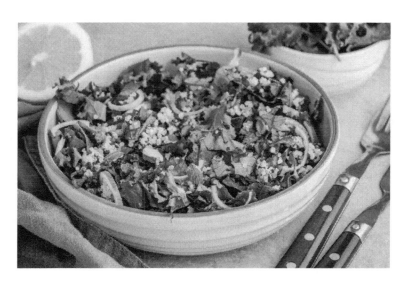

## Ingredients:

- 2 cups kale; remove stems
- 2 tbsp lemon juice
- ½ tbsp olive oil
- ¼ cup almonds, sliced
- ½ cup cooked quinoa
- For dressing:
- ¼ cup Tahini

- ½ tsp garlic powder
- 3 tbsp warm water
- 2 tbsp lemon juice
- ½ tsp sea salt

## Directions:

- In a small bowl, whisk together all dressing ingredients until well combined. Set aside.
- In a large bowl, mix together kale, olive oil, and lemon juice.
- Add quinoa and almonds and mix well with kale.
- Pour dressing over salad and toss well.
- Serve and enjoy.

## Nutritional value (amount per serving):

- Calories 476
- Fat 28.4g
- Carbohydrates 44.3g
- Sugar 1.5g
- Protein 16g
- Cholesterol 0mg

# 3 - Spinach & Strawberry Salad with Balsamic Vinaigrette

**Preparation time: 10 minutes**

**Cooking time: 5 minutes**

**Serves: 4**

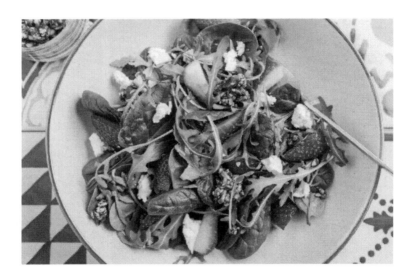

## Ingredients:

- 16oz strawberries, sliced
- 16oz spinach
- ½ cup pecans, chopped
- ½ cup goat cheese, crumbled
- For dressing:
- 1/3 cup balsamic vinegar
- ½ cup olive oil

- 1 tsp Dijon mustard
- 2 tsp maple syrup
- Pepper
- Salt

## Directions:

- In a small bowl, whisk together all dressing ingredients and set aside.
- In a mixing bowl, mix together strawberries, spinach, pecans, and goat cheese.
- Pour dressing over salad and toss well.
- Serve and enjoy.

## Nutritional value (amount per serving):

- Calories 355
- Fat 31.3g
- Carbohydrates 15.8g
- Sugar 8.4g
- Protein 7.7g
- Cholesterol 12mg

# 4 - Greek Salad with Feta & Olives

**Preparation time: 10 minutes**

**Cooking time: 5 minutes**

**Serves: 4**

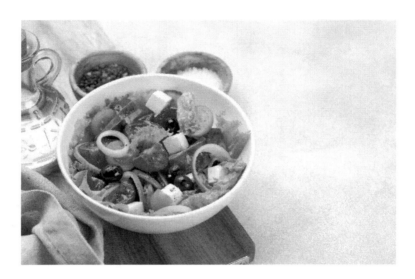

## Ingredients:

- 6 cups romaine lettuce, chopped
- 1 cup feta cheese, crumbled
- 1 cup olives, pitted
- 2 cups cucumber, sliced
- 1 cup cherry tomatoes, sliced
- 1 red bell pepper, chopped
- For dressing:
- ¼ cup olive oil
- 2 tsp dried oregano

- 2 tsp garlic, crushed
- 2 tbsp lemon juice
- 2 tbsp red wine vinegar
- Pepper
- Salt

## Directions:

- In a large bowl, mix together lettuce, olives, cucumber, tomatoes, and bell pepper.
- Add crumbled cheese on top.
- In a small bowl, whisk together all dressing ingredients and pour over salad.
- Serve and enjoy.

## Nutritional value (amount per serving):

- Calories 290
- Fat 24.7g
- Carbohydrates 13.2g
- Sugar 6.1g
- Protein 7.3g
- Cholesterol 33mg

# 5 - Roasted Vegetable Salad with Turmeric Dressing

**Preparation time: 10 minutes**

**Cooking time: 30 minutes**

**Serves: 4**

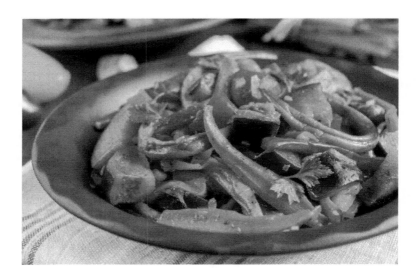

## Ingredients:

- 1 medium sweet potato, peeled & diced into chunks
- 1 medium zucchini, diced
- 1 medium eggplant, diced into chunks
- 1 medium onion, quartered
- 2 bell peppers, cored & diced
- For dressing:

- 3 tbsp olive oil
- ½ tsp cumin powder
- ½ tsp chili powder
- 1 tsp garlic powder
- 1 tsp turmeric
- Pepper
- Salt

**Directions:**

- In a small bowl, whisk together all dressing ingredients and set aside.
- Add sweet potatoes, zucchini, eggplant, onion, and bell peppers into the large mixing bowl.
- Pour dressing over salad and toss until well coated.
- Spread veggies onto a baking sheet and roast at 425F for 35 minutes. Turn veggies halfway through.
- Serve and enjoy.

**Nutritional value (amount per serving):**

- Calories 189
- Fat 11.2g
- Carbohydrates 22.5g
- Sugar 10.5g
- Protein 3.4g
- Cholesterol 0mg

# 6 - Beetroot & Arugula Salad with Citrus Dressing

**Preparation time: 10 minutes**

**Cooking time: 5 minutes**

**Serves: 4**

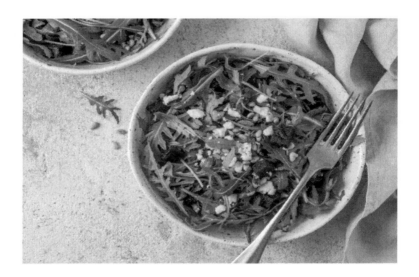

## Ingredients:

- 4 medium beets, roasted & cut into bite-size pieces
- 8 cups baby arugula
- 1 shallot, sliced
- ¼ cup walnuts, toasted & chopped
- For dressing:
- 2 tbsp orange juice

- ½ cup olive oil
- ½ tsp maple syrup
- ½ tbsp Dijon mustard
- 1 tbsp lemon juice
- Pepper
- Salt

## Directions:

- In a small bowl, whisk together all dressing ingredients and set aside.
- Place the arugula on a serving plate. Top with beet, shallot, and walnuts.
- Drizzle with dressing and serve.

## Nutritional value (amount per serving):

- Calories 328
- Fat 30.4g
- Carbohydrates 14.2g
- Sugar 10.1g
- Protein 4.8g
- Cholesterol 0mg

# 7 - Avocado & Mango Salad with Lime Cilantro Dressing

**Preparation time: 10 minutes**

**Cooking time: 5 minutes**

**Serves: 8**

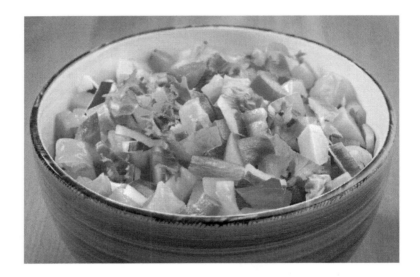

## Ingredients:

- 2 large mangos, diced
- 1 avocado, diced
- 2 tbsp fresh basil, chopped
- 2 tbsp fresh mint, chopped
- ¼ cup cilantro, chopped
- 1 cup cucumber, diced
- ½ cup onion, diced

- 1 red bell pepper, diced
- 1 tbsp olive oil
- 2 tbsp maple syrup
- ¼ cup lime juice
- ½ tsp salt

## Directions:

- In a small bowl, whisk together lime juice, olive oil, maple syrup, and salt. Set aside.
- In a mixing bowl, mix together mango, basil, mint, cilantro, avocado, cucumber, onion, and bell pepper.
- Pour the lime mixture over the salad and toss well.
- Serve and enjoy.

## Nutritional value (amount per serving):

- Calories 115
- Fat 6.9g
- Carbohydrates 14.2g
- Sugar 10g
- Protein 1.2g
- Cholesterol 0mg

# 8 - Quinoa & Chickpea Salad with Roasted Vegetables

**Preparation time: 10 minutes**

**Cooking time: 25 minutes**

**Serves: 4**

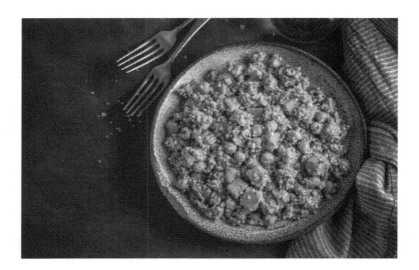

## Ingredients:

- 1 ½ cups cooked quinoa
- 15oz can chickpeas, drained & rinsed
- ½ tsp dried oregano
- 1 tsp garlic powder
- 2 tbsp olive oil
- 8oz mushrooms, sliced
- 1 medium sweet potato, cut into ½-inch cubes

- 1 yellow bell pepper, cut into chunks
- 1 medium onion, cut into chunks
- Pepper
- Salt

## Directions:

- Preheat the oven to 400F.
- Place veggies and chickpeas onto a parchment-lined baking sheet.
- Drizzle with olive oil and sprinkle with oregano, garlic powder, pepper, and salt.
- Bake in preheated oven for 20-25 minutes. Stir veggies halfway through.
- In a mixing bowl, add cooked quinoa and roasted veggies and mix well.
- Serve and enjoy.

## Nutritional value (amount per serving):

- Calories 483
- Fat 12.4g
- Carbohydrates 78.2g
- Sugar 5.7g
- Protein 17.4g
- Cholesterol 0mg

# 9 - Cucumber & Tomato Salad with Yogurt Dressing

**Preparation time: 10 minutes**

**Cooking time: 5 minutes**

**Serves: 6**

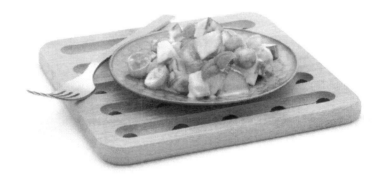

## Ingredients:

- 6 cups tomatoes, cut into chunks
- ¼ cup Greek yogurt
- ½ cup mayonnaise
- ½ cup fresh herbs, chopped
- ½ medium onion, sliced
- 1 cucumber, chopped
- 1 tsp kosher salt

## Directions:

- In a large bowl, mix together yogurt, mayonnaise, and salt until smooth.
- Add tomatoes, fresh herbs, onion, and cucumber to the yogurt mixture and mix until well-coated.
- Serve and enjoy.

## Nutritional value (amount per serving):

- Calories 133
- Fat 7.3g
- Carbohydrates 16.4g
- Sugar 7.6g
- Protein 3.4g
- Cholesterol 6mg

# 10 - Broccoli & Cranberry Salad with Poppy Seed Dressing

**Preparation time: 10 minutes**

**Cooking time: 5 minutes**

**Serves: 6**

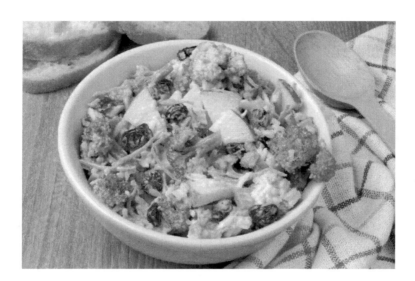

## Ingredients:

- 1lb broccoli, cut into florets
- ½ cup dried cranberries
- ½ cup pumpkin seeds
- ½lb cabbage, shredded
- 10 Brussels sprouts, sliced
- 2 tbsp apple cider vinegar
- ½ cup Greek yogurt

- 1 tbsp poppy seeds
- 1 tbsp honey
- Salt

## Directions:

- In a small bowl, whisk together yogurt, honey, poppy seeds, vinegar, and salt.
- In a large bowl, mix together broccoli, cranberries, pumpkin seeds, cabbage, and Brussels sprouts.
- Pour dressing over salad and stir well to coat.
- Cover and place in refrigerator for 30 minutes.
- Serve and enjoy.

## Nutritional value (amount per serving):

- Calories 148
- Fat 6.7g
- Carbohydrates 16.9g
- Sugar 7.4g
- Protein 8.5g
- Cholesterol 1mg

# 11 - Watermelon & Feta Salad with Mint Lime Dressing

**Preparation time: 10 minutes**

**Cooking time: 5 minutes**

**Serves: 4**

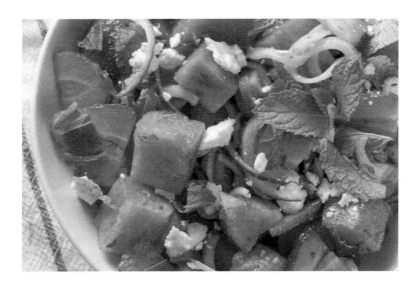

## Ingredients:

- 3lbs watermelon, remove seeds & cut into 1-inch cubes
- 12 fresh mint leaves, chopped
- 8oz feta cheese, crumbled
- For dressing:
- 1/3 cup olive oil
- 2 fresh lime juice

- Pepper
- Salt

## Directions:

- In a small bowl, whisk together all dressing ingredients and set aside.
- In a large bowl, add watermelon, crumbled cheese, and mint leaves and toss well.
- Drizzle the dressing over the salad and serve.

## Nutritional value (amount per serving):

- Calories 417
- Fat 29.6g
- Carbohydrates 32.6g
- Sugar 23.6g
- Protein 11.3g
- Cholesterol 50mg

# 12 - Arugula & Pomegranate Salad with Toasted Pecans

**Preparation time: 10 minutes**

**Cooking time: 5 minutes**

**Serves: 4**

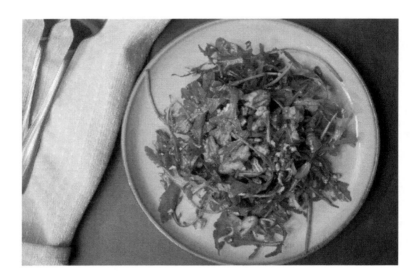

## Ingredients:

- 5 oz baby arugula
- 1/3 cup pecans, toasted & chopped
- ½ cup pomegranate seeds
- For dressing:
- ¼ cup olive oil
- 2 tbsp lemon juice
- 1 garlic clove, minced

- ¼ tsp pepper
- ¼ tsp salt

## Directions:

- In a small bowl, whisk together olive oil, lemon juice, garlic, pepper, and salt.
- In a mixing bowl, mix together arugula, pecans, and pomegranate seeds.
- Drizzle dressing over salad and toss well.
- Serve and enjoy.

## Nutritional value (amount per serving):

- Calories 141
- Fat 13.7g
- Carbohydrates 5g
- Sugar 2.4g
- Protein 1.3g
- Cholesterol 0mg

# 13 - Asian Cabbage Slaw with Ginger Sesame Dressing

**Preparation time: 10 minutes**

**Cooking time: 5 minutes**

**Serves: 8**

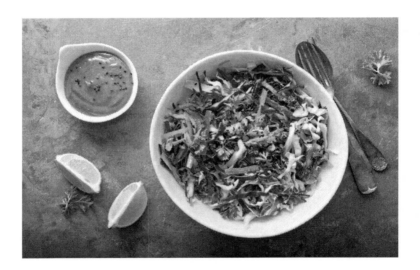

## Ingredients:

- 2 cups red cabbage, shredded
- 2 carrots, julienned
- 3 cups green cabbage, shredded
- ½ cup fresh mint, chopped
- ½ cup cilantro, chopped
- 3 green onions, sliced
- 3 cups beansprouts

- For dressing:
- 1 tbsp ginger, grated
- 1 tsp sesame oil
- 1 ½ tbsp honey
- 3 tbsp soy sauce, low-sodium
- 2 tbsp oyster sauce
- 3 tbsp rice wine vinegar
- 2 tbsp olive oil
- 1 garlic clove, minced
- ½ tsp salt

## Directions:

- In a small bowl, mix together all dressing ingredients and set aside.
- In a large bowl, mix together red cabbage, carrots, green cabbage, mint, cilantro, green onions, and beansprouts.
- Pour dressing over salad and toss well.
- Serve and enjoy.

## Nutritional value (amount per serving):

- Calories 141
- Fat 13.7g
- Carbohydrates 5g
- Sugar 2.4g
- Protein 1.3g
- Cholesterol 0mg

# 14 - Quinoa & Black Bean Salad Lime Dressing

**Preparation time: 10 minutes**

**Cooking time: 5 minutes**

**Serves: 8**

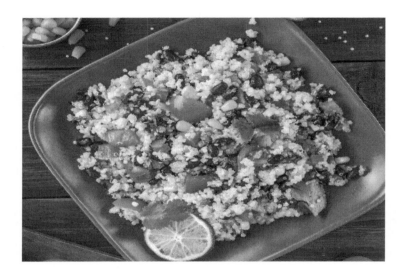

**Ingredients:**

- 3 cups cooked quinoa
- ¼ cup green onions, chopped
- 1 avocado, diced
- ¼ cup sweetcorn
- 2 cups cherry tomatoes, cut in half
- 14 oz can black beans, drained & rinsed
- For dressing:

- ¼ cup olive oil
- 2 tbsp cilantro, chopped
- ¼ tsp cayenne
- ½ tsp paprika
- 1 lime juice
- Pepper
- Salt

## Directions:

- In a large bowl, mix together quinoa, green onions, avocado, cherry tomatoes, and black beans.
- In a small bowl, mix together all dressing ingredients and pour over salad.
- Toss well and serve.

## Nutritional value (amount per serving):

- Calories 400
- Fat 15.4g
- Carbohydrates 54.9g
- Sugar 1.9g
- Protein 12.8g
- Cholesterol 0mg

# 15 - Roasted Sweet Potato & Kale Salad with Dijon Dressing

**Preparation time: 10 minutes**

**Cooking time: 25 minutes**

**Serves: 4**

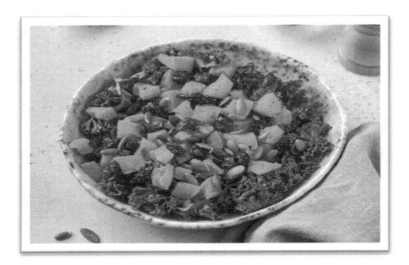

## Ingredients:

- 1 large sweet potato, peeled & cut into cubes
- 1/3 cup pumpkin seeds, toasted
- 4 large kale leaves, chopped
- ½ tbsp olive oil
- ¾ cup cranberries
- ¼ tsp salt
- For dressing:
- 1 tbsp maple syrup

- 1 tbsp Dijon mustard
- 3 tbsp olive oil
- 2 tbsp white wine vinegar
- Pepper
- Salt

## Directions:

- Preheat the oven to 400F.
- In a bowl, toss sweet potato with oil and salt.
- Spread sweet potato onto a parchment-lined baking sheet and bake in preheated oven for 10 minutes.
- Mix cranberries with sweet potatoes and cook for 10 minutes more.
- In a large bowl, add kale, sweet potatoes, pumpkin seeds, and cranberries. Mix well.
- In a small bowl, whisk together all dressing ingredients and pour over salad.
- Toss well and serve.

## Nutritional value (amount per serving):

- Calories 270
- Fat 17.8g
- Carbohydrates 23.9g
- Sugar 6.8g
- Protein 5.9g
- Cholesterol 0mg

# Chapter 5 – Main Dish Recipes

## The Place of the Main Dish in the Anti-Inflammatory Diet

The main food in an anti-inflammatory diet is really important because it is the core part of your meal and helps to support your overall health and well-being. The main dish lets you add healthy foods to your meals. Usually, it has a type of lean protein like chicken, fish, beans, or tofu. These proteins are really important for making muscles bigger, fixing them when they get hurt, and keeping your body healthy. They also give you important amino acids, vitamins, and minerals.

An anti-inflammatory diet relies on the main dish to incorporate anti-inflammatory components, including vegetables, wholegrains, herbs, spices, and healthy fats. Antioxidants and phytochemicals in leafy greens, cruciferous vegetables such as broccoli, cauliflower, etc, and colorful food, fight inflammation. Quinoa and brown rice are fiber-rich are anti-inflammatory. Turmeric, ginger, garlic, and oregano are also anti-inflammatory ingredients. Olive oil, avocados, almonds, and seeds provide anti-inflammatory fats.

The main course, when served with side dishes like vegetables, wholegrains, and healthy fats, helps make a well-rounded and healthy meal. This mix of foods helps you get different important nutrients, antioxidants, fiber, and other good substances that help with your overall health and decrease inflammation. The main dish can be changed according to different diets, like vegetarian, gluten-free, or dairy-free. People can customize their meals and include ingredients that help reduce inflammation.

When you make the main dish with ingredients that fight inflammation, it can help decrease inflammation in your body. Long-term inflammation is linked to different health problems like diabetes, heart disease, and some types of cancer. Eating anti-inflammatory main dishes regularly helps keep you healthy and lowers the chance of getting long-term illnesses.

# 1 - Baked Salmon with Lemon & Dill

**Preparation time: 10 minutes**

**Cooking time: 20 minutes**

**Serves: 4**

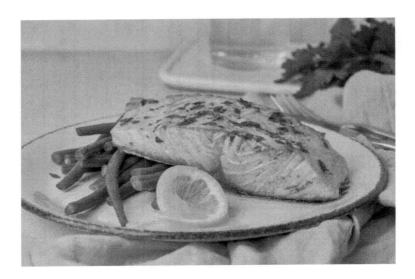

## Ingredients:

- 1 ¼lbs salmon fillets
- 1 tbsp lemon juice
- 2 tbsp olive oil
- 1 tbsp dill, chopped
- 3 garlic cloves, minced
- Pepper
- Salt

## Directions:

- Preheat the oven to 350F.
- Season salmon fillets with pepper and salt and place into the baking dish.
- In a small bowl, mix together olive oil, lemon juice, dill, and garlic and pour over salmon fillets.
- Bake in preheated oven for 15-20 minutes.
- Serve and enjoy.

## Nutritional value (amount per serving):

- Calories 254
- Fat 15.8g
- Carbohydrates 1.3g
- Sugar 0.1g
- Protein 27.8g
- Cholesterol 63mg

# 2 - Turmeric Chicken Stir-Fry

**Preparation time: 10 minutes**

**Cooking time: 10 minutes**

**Serves: 2**

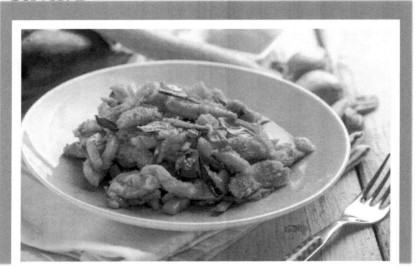

## Ingredients:

- 12oz chicken breast, boneless & cut into bite-size pieces
- 2 garlic cloves, minced
- 1 cup shredded carrots
- 2 cups broccoli florets
- 1 tbsp olive oil
- ¼ tsp ground coriander
- ¼ tsp ground ginger
- 1 tsp ground turmeric

- Pepper
- Salt

## Directions:

- In a large bowl, mix together chicken, turmeric, coriander, ginger, pepper, and salt until well coated.
- Heat oil in a pan over high heat.
- Once the oil is hot then add chicken to the pan and cook for 3-5 minutes on each side. Transfer chicken to a plate and set aside.
- Add carrots and broccoli to the same pan and stir-fry for 3-4 minutes.
- Return chicken to the pan along with garlic and cook for 2 minutes.
- Serve and enjoy.

## Nutritional value (amount per serving):

- Calories 317
- Fat 11.7g
- Carbohydrates 13.3g
- Sugar 4.3g
- Protein 39.4g
- Cholesterol 109mg

# 3 - Lentil & Vegetable Curry

**Preparation time: 10 minutes**

**Cooking time: 20 minutes**

**Serves: 6**

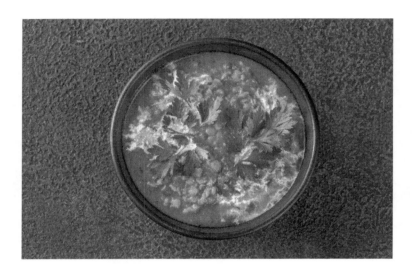

## Ingredients:

- 15oz can lentils, drained & rinsed
- 3 cups baby spinach
- 1 lime juice
- 2 tsp maple syrup
- 1 tbsp cornstarch
- 2 tbsp red curry paste
- 14 oz can coconut milk
- 1 red bell pepper, seeded & chopped
- 2 medium carrots, peeled & chopped

- 2 cups broccoli florets
- 2 cups cauliflower florets
- 1 medium sweet potato, peeled & cubed
- 2 tbsp curry powder
- 1 tbsp ginger, grated
- 3 garlic cloves, minced
- 1 medium onion, chopped
- 1 tbsp olive oil
- Salt

**Directions:**

- Heat oil in a large pot over medium heat.
- Add onion and sauté for 2-3 minutes.
- Add ginger and garlic and cook for 1 minute.
- Add curry powder and sauté for 1-2 minutes.
- Add sweet potato, lentils, red pepper, carrots, broccoli, and cauliflower to the pot and stir well.
- Add curry paste, coconut milk, and salt and stir well. Bring to a boil, turn heat to low and simmer for 10 minutes or until sweet potatoes are tender.
- In a small bowl, whisk together cornstarch and 2 tablespoons water, then stir into the lentil curry to thicken.
- Add maple syrup, spinach, and lime juice and cook until spinach is wilted. Season with salt.
- Serve and enjoy.

## Nutritional value (amount per serving):

- Calories 318
- Fat 21g
- Carbohydrates 29.6g
- Sugar 9.2g
- Protein 7.5g
- Cholesterol 2mg

# 4 - Quinoa Stuffed Bell Peppers

**Preparation time: 10 minutes**

**Cooking time: 25 minutes**

**Serves: 6**

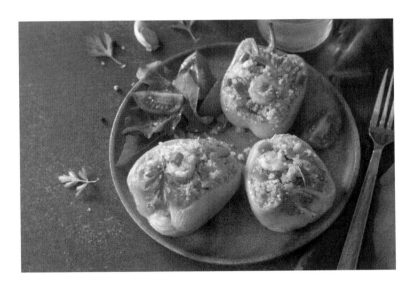

## Ingredients:

- 3 bell peppers, cut in half & seeds removed
- 2 tbsp harissa
- ¼ cup feta cheese, crumbled
- ½ cup cherry tomatoes, sliced
- 1/3 cup can chickpeas, rinsed
- ½ tsp oregano
- 2 garlic cloves, minced
- 1 ½ cups cooked quinoa

- ½ tsp salt

## Directions:

- Preheat the oven to 400F.
- In a bowl, mix together quinoa, tomatoes, chickpeas, oregano, garlic, and salt.
- Stuff the quinoa mixture into each bell pepper half.
- Place stuffed peppers onto a baking sheet and bake in preheated oven for 20-25 minutes.
- Top peppers with cheese and drizzle with harissa paste.
- Serve and enjoy.

## Nutritional value (amount per serving):

- Calories 229
- Fat 5.1g
- Carbohydrates 38g
- Sugar 5g
- Protein 8.7g
- Cholesterol 7mg

# 5 - Grilled Shrimp & Vegetable Skewers

**Preparation time: 10 minutes**

**Cooking time: 10 minutes**

**Serves: 8**

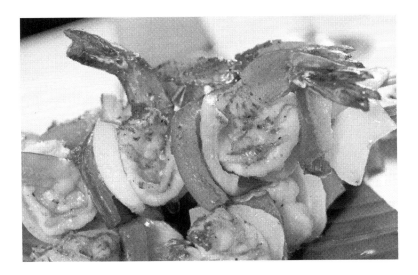

## Ingredients:

- 2lbs shrimp, thawed
- 1 large onion, cut into 1-inch pieces
- 2 bell peppers, cut into 1-inch pieces
- 2 small zucchini, sliced
- For marinade:
- 1 tbsp onion, minced
- 2 garlic cloves, minced
- 2 tbsp red wine vinegar
- 1 tbsp lime juice

- ¾ cup olive oil
- ¼ cup fresh oregano, minced
- 1 cup parsley, minced
- Pepper
- Salt

## Directions:

- Add all marinade ingredients into the large mixing bowl and mix well.
- Add shrimp, bell pepper, onion, and zucchini to the marinade and mix until well coated. Cover and place in refrigerator for 30 minutes.
- Preheat the grill to high heat.
- Thread shrimp and vegetables onto the skewers.
- Place skewers on a hot grill and cook for 10 minutes. Flip halfway through.
- Serve and enjoy.

## Nutritional value (amount per serving):

- Calories 332
- Fat 21.3g
- Carbohydrates 9.5g
- Sugar 3.1g
- Protein 27.3g
- Cholesterol 239mg

# 6 - Mediterranean Baked Chicken

**Preparation time: 10 minutes**

**Cooking time: 30 minutes**

**Serves: 4**

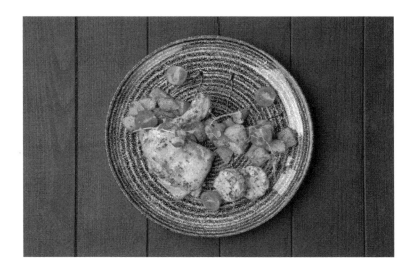

## Ingredients:

- 8 chicken thighs
- 4 tbsp capers
- 3oz olives, pitted
- 14oz cherry tomatoes
- 1 cup chicken stock
- 4 garlic cloves, crushed
- 2 tbsp olive oil
- Pepper

- Salt

## Directions:

- Preheat the oven to 390F.
- Brush chicken with olive oil and season with pepper and salt.
- Place chicken into the oven-safe pan and cook over medium heat for 10 minutes.
- Add garlic and chicken stock and cook for 3-5 minutes. Remove pan from heat.
- Add capers, olives, tomatoes, pepper, and salt, and mix well with chicken.
- Place pan in preheated oven and bake for 15-20 minutes or until chicken is cooked.
- Serve and enjoy.

## Nutritional value (amount per serving):

- Calories 666
- Fat 31.3g
- Carbohydrates 6.8g
- Sugar 2.9g
- Protein 86.1g
- Cholesterol 260mg

# 7 - Spaghetti Squash with Tomato & Basil Sauce

**Preparation time: 10 minutes**

**Cooking time: 15 minutes**

**Serves: 4**

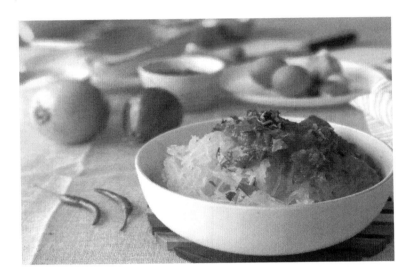

## Ingredients:

- 1 large spaghetti squash, cut in half & seeds scooped out
- ½ cup basil, sliced
- 1½ tsp garlic, minced
- 2 tbsp olive oil
- 2¼lbs tomatoes, chopped
- Pepper

- Salt

**Directions:**

- In a mixing bowl, toss tomatoes with garlic, oil, basil, pepper, and salt and set aside for 15 minutes.
- Meanwhile, place spaghetti squash in a microwave-safe dish and cook on high power for 15 minutes.
- Using a fork, scrape spaghetti squash from the peel, add to bowl with tomato mixture, and toss to coat.
- Serve and enjoy.

**Nutritional value (amount per serving):**

- Calories 116
- Fat 7.7g
- Carbohydrates 12.1g
- Sugar 6.7g
- Protein 2.6g
- Cholesterol 0mg

# 8 - Moroccan Chickpea Stew

**Preparation time: 10 minutes**

**Cooking time: 30 minutes**

**Serves: 4**

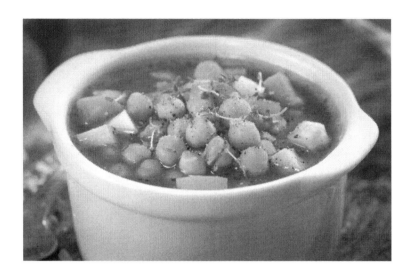

## Ingredients:

- 15oz can chickpeas, drained
- 2 cups kale, chopped
- 1 tbsp maple syrup
- 1/8 tsp cayenne
- ½ tsp turmeric
- ½ tsp cinnamon
- 1 tsp paprika
- 2 tsp curry powder
- 1½ tsp cumin

- 1 cup vegetable broth
- 2 cups crushed tomatoes
- 2 medium sweet potatoes, peeled & cut into cubes
- 4 garlic cloves, chopped
- 1 tbsp olive oil
- 1 onion, chopped
- Pepper
- Salt

## Directions:

- Heat olive oil in a large pot over medium-high heat.
- Add garlic and onion and sauté for 1-2 minutes.
- Add chickpeas and sweet potatoes and mix well.
- Add crushed tomatoes, broth, maple syrup, spices, and salt, and stir everything well. Bring to boil.
- Turn heat to low, cover and simmer for 20-30 minutes or until sweet potatoes are tender.
- Add kale and stir until kale is wilted.
- Serve and enjoy.

## Nutritional value (amount per serving):

- Calories 359
- Fat 5.7g
- Carbohydrates 67.3g
- Sugar 11.9g
- Protein 12.5g
- Cholesterol 0mg

# 9 - Grilled Tofu with Balsamic Glaze

**Preparation time: 10 minutes**

**Cooking time: 10 minutes**

**Serves: 4**

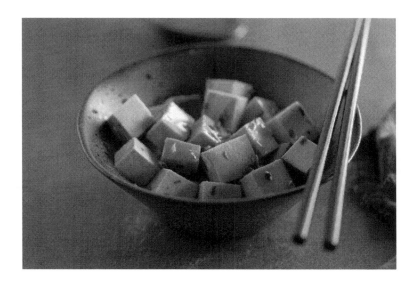

## Ingredients:

- 16oz tofu, pressed, drained & cut into ½-inch thick slices
- 2 tbsp olive oil
- 2 tbsp water
- 2 tbsp maple syrup
- 2 tbsp balsamic vinegar
- ½ tsp salt

## Directions:

- In a bowl, mix together balsamic vinegar, maple syrup, water, oil, and salt.
- Add tofu and mix until well coated. Cover and place in refrigerator for 30 minutes.
- Preheat the grill to medium heat.
- Arrange marinated tofu slices onto a hot grill and cook for 5 minutes on each side.
- Serve and enjoy.

## Nutritional value (amount per serving):

- Calories 167
- Fat 11.8g
- Carbohydrates 8.7g
- Sugar 6.7g
- Protein 9.3g
- Cholesterol 0mg

# 10 - Cauliflower Fried Rice

## Preparation time: 10 minutes

## Cooking time: 10 minutes

## Serves: 6

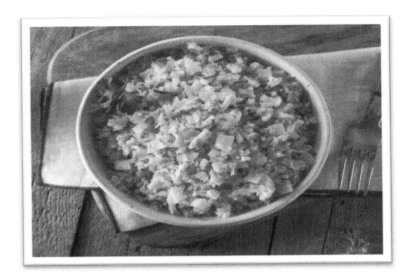

## Ingredients:

- 2 eggs
- 3 cups cauliflower rice
- 1 green onion, diced
- 2 tbsp coconut aminos
- 1 tsp garlic powder
- 1 ½ cups cooked chicken, diced
- 1 cup carrots, chopped
- ½ cup peas

- 1 onion, diced
- 2 tbsp sesame oil
- Pepper
- Salt

## Directions:

- Heat sesame oil in a pan over medium heat.
- Add onion, carrots, and peas and sauté for 5-7 minutes or until vegetables are soft.
- Add egg and stir until cooked.
- Add chicken, coconut aminos, cauliflower rice, garlic powder, pepper, and salt and stir well and cook for 2-3 minutes.
- Garnish with green onions and serve.

## Nutritional value (amount per serving):

- Calories 174
- Fat 8g
- Carbohydrates 10.3g
- Sugar 4.6g
- Protein 15.1g
- Cholesterol 82mg

# 11 - Zucchini Noodles with Turkey Meatballs

**Preparation time: 10 minutes**

**Cooking time: 35 minutes**

**Serves: 4**

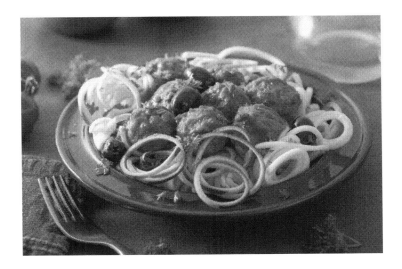

## Ingredients:

- 4 medium zucchini, spiralized
- 1 garlic clove, minced
- 24oz marinara sauce
- 2 tbsp olive oil
- 1 large egg
- ¼ cup Parmesan cheese, grated
- ½ cup wholewheat breadcrumbs

- ½ cup cottage cheese
- 1lb ground turkey
- Pepper
- Salt

## Directions:

- Heat 1 tablespoon of olive oil in a pan over medium heat.
- Add zucchini noodles and sauté for 4-5 minutes. Season with pepper and salt.
- Transfer zucchini noodles onto a plate.
- Heat remaining oil in the same pan.
- In a bowl, mix together ground turkey, egg, Parmesan cheese, breadcrumbs, cottage cheese, pepper, and salt until well combined.
- Make equally-shaped of balls from meat mixture and add into the pan and cook over medium-high heat for 4-5 minutes or until lightly brown on all sides.
- Add marinara sauce, cover and simmer for 5 minutes or until meatballs are cooked.
- Top the zucchini noodles with meatballs.
- Serve and enjoy.

## Nutritional value (amount per serving):

- Calories 537
- Fat 28g
- Carbohydrates 34.3g
- Sugar 18.6g
- Protein 44.1g
- Cholesterol 172mg

# 12 - Sweet Potato Black Bean Enchiladas

**Preparation time: 10 minutes**

**Cooking time: 60 minutes**

**Serves: 8**

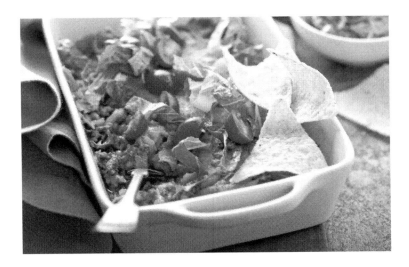

## Ingredients:

- 2 sweet potatoes, peeled, thinly sliced & boiled until tender
- 1/3 cup cilantro, chopped
- 2 cups low-fat Mexican cheese blend, shredded
- 2 cups cooked chicken breast, shredded
- 15oz can black beans, drained & rinsed
- 2 cups enchilada sauce

- 3 cups spinach, chopped
- 2 red bell peppers, diced
- 1 onion, diced
- 1 tbsp olive oil

## Directions:

- Preheat the oven to 375F.
- Heat olive oil in a pan over medium-high heat.
- Add onion and bell pepper and sauté until tender.
- Add spinach and sauté until spinach wilted.
- Spread half enchilada sauce in greased 9x13-inch baking dish.
- Arrange half-sweet of the potato slices over the enchilada sauce. Sprinkle half of the black beans, chicken, and sautéed vegetables.
- Top with 1 cup of cheese. Repeat these layers.
- Cover the dish with foil and bake in preheated oven for 40 minutes. Remove the cover and bake for 5-10 minutes.
- Garnish with cilantro and serve.

## Nutritional value (amount per serving):

- Calories 228
- Fat 5.1g
- Carbohydrates 30.6g
- Sugar 3g
- Protein 17.4g
- Cholesterol 22mg

# 13 - Eggplant & Chickpea Tagine

**Preparation time: 10 minutes**

**Cooking time: 40 minutes**

**Serves: 4**

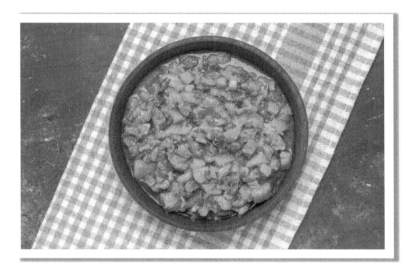

## Ingredients:

- 2 small eggplants, cut into 1-inch pieces
- 2½ cups vegetable stock
- ½ cup dried apricots
- 14oz can chickpeas
- 14oz can tomatoes, chopped
- ½ tsp cinnamon
- 2 tbsp Moroccan spice blend
- 1 red pepper, diced
- 1 medium courgette, cut into 1-inch pieces

- 3 garlic cloves
- 3 tbsp olive oil
- 1 onion, diced
- Pepper
- Salt

**Directions:**

- Heat 2 tablespoons of olive oil in a large pan over medium heat.
- Add eggplant pieces and cook until slightly golden. Remove eggplant pieces from the pan and set aside.
- Heat remaining oil in the same pan.
- Add onion and sauté for 2-3 minutes. Add garlic and sauté for 30 seconds.
- Add red pepper and courgette and cook for 5-6 minutes.
- Add Moroccan spice and cinnamon and stir well.
- Add tomatoes, apricots, chickpeas, and stock. Stir well and bring to a simmer.
- Add eggplant pieces and stir well.
- Cover pan with lid. Bake in preheated oven at 375F for 25 minutes or until vegetables are tender. Remove pan from oven
- Serve and enjoy.

**Nutritional value (amount per serving):**

- Calories 352
- Fat 13.4g
- Carbohydrates 53.1g
- Sugar 16g
- Protein 9.9g
- Cholesterol 0mg

# 14 - Quinoa & Spinach Stuffed Portobello Mushrooms

**Preparation time: 10 minutes**

**Cooking time: 23 minutes**

**Serves: 4**

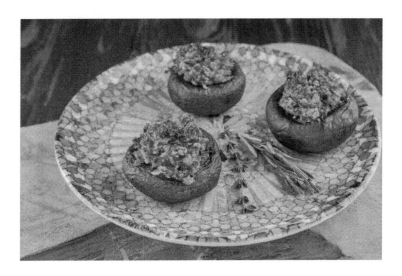

## Ingredients:

- 1 cup cooked quinoa
- ½ cup mozzarella cheese, shredded
- 4 large portobello mushrooms, rinsed; remove stem & using a spoon, scrape out the gills
- ½ tsp dried thyme
- ½ tsp dried oregano
- 1 tsp dried parsley

- 1 tbsp lemon juice
- ½ cup Parmesan cheese, grated
- 6oz spinach, cleaned & stemmed
- 1 tsp garlic, minced
- 4 tbsp olive oil
- ½ cup onion, diced
- Pepper
- Salt

## Directions:

- Preheat the oven to 350F.
- Heat 2 tablespoons of olive oil in a pan over medium heat.
- Add onion and sauté for 2-3 minutes. Add garlic and sauté for 30 seconds.
- Add spinach and cook until spinach is completely wilted. Turn off the heat.
- Add quinoa, lemon juice, dried herbs, Parmesan cheese, pepper, and salt, and mix well.
- Brush the outside of the mushrooms with oil.
- Stuff quinoa spinach mixture into each mushroom cavity and sprinkle each with mozzarella cheese.
- Place stuffed mushrooms onto a parchment-lined baking sheet and bake in preheated oven for 20 minutes.
- Serve and enjoy.

## Nutritional value (amount per serving):

- Calories 339
- Fat 18.4g
- Carbohydrates 35.3g
- Sugar 2.4g
- Protein 11.8g
- Cholesterol 4mg

# 15 - Baked Cod with Herb Crust

**Preparation time: 10 minutes**

**Cooking time: 15 minutes**

**Serves: 4**

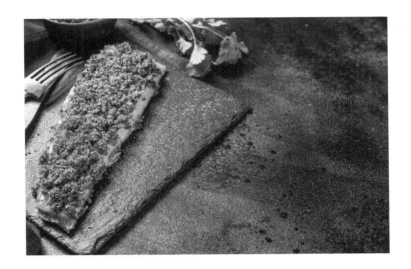

## Ingredients:

- 4 cod fillets
- 1 tbsp olive oil
- 2½ oz wholewheat breadcrumbs
- 1 lemon zest
- 1 tbsp parsley, chopped
- 1 tbsp chives, chopped
- 1 tbsp thyme, chopped
- 1 tbsp rosemary, chopped
- Pepper

- Salt

## Directions:

- Preheat the oven to 400F.
- In a small bowl, mix together breadcrumbs, herbs, lemon zest, olive oil, pepper, and salt.
- Arrange cod fillets onto a parchment-lined baking sheet.
- Spread breadcrumb mixture on top of each cod fillet and bake in preheated oven for 10-15 minutes.
- Serve and enjoy.

## Nutritional value (amount per serving):

- Calories 195
- Fat 7.8g
- Carbohydrates 15g
- Sugar 0.1g
- Protein 22.1g
- Cholesterol 55mg

# Chapter 6 - Side Dish Recipes

## The Place of Side Dish in the Anti-Inflammatory Diet

Side dishes play an important role in an anti-inflammatory diet because of the flavor, diversity, and health benefits that are added to the main course. A balanced, nutrient-rich dinner requires side dishes. Vitamin, mineral, antioxidant, and fiber-rich vegetables, wholegrains, legumes, and salads are common. These nutrients improve general health, reduce inflammation, and boost your immune system. Antioxidants and phytochemicals in vegetables, especially leafy greens, and colorful ones, fight inflammation and oxidative stress. Complex carbs, fiber, and minerals in wholegrains regulate blood sugar and satiety. Beans and lentils provide protein, fiber, and minerals. Side dishes provide a diversified dietary profile for good health.

Side dishes lend flavor, variety, and depth to a meal. They enhance the overall dining experience by introducing new flavors, sensations, and culinary components. By incorporating a diversity of side dishes, monotonous meals can be avoided and adherence to an anti-inflammatory diet can be increased. Side dishes are an excellent opportunity to include anti-inflammatory ingredients in your diet. Many side dishes feature wholegrains, vegetables, herbs, spices, and healthy fats that come with anti-inflammatory properties.

Meals that include anti-inflammatory side dishes encourage long-term health benefits. Numerous illnesses, including heart-related disease, obesity, and several cancers, are linked to chronic inflammation. You may provide your body with the resources it needs to fight inflammation and lower your risk of developing certain chronic diseases by frequently including side dishes that are abundant in anti-inflammatory substances.

Side dishes provide options for accommodating various dietary preferences and restrictions. They can be changed to fit different ways of eating, like vegan, vegetarian, gluten-free, or no-dairy diets. This flexibility lets people customize their meals while still following the guidelines of a diet that reduces inflammation.

# 1 - Roasted Broccoli with Garlic & Lemon

**Preparation time: 10 minutes**

**Cooking time: 10 minutes**

**Serves: 4**

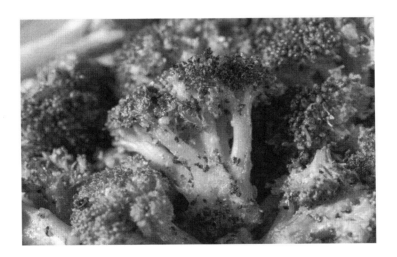

## Ingredients:

- 12oz broccoli florets
- ½ lemon juice
- 2 garlic cloves, minced
- 1 tbsp olive oil
- Pepper
- Salt

## Directions:

- Preheat the oven to 400F.
- In a bowl, toss broccoli with oil, lemon juice, garlic, pepper, and salt.
- Spread broccoli florets onto a parchment-lined baking sheet and bake in preheated oven for 10 minutes or until tender.
- Serve and enjoy.

## Nutritional value (amount per serving):

- Calories 63
- Fat 3.8g
- Carbohydrates 6.3g
- Sugar 1.6g
- Protein 2.5g
- Cholesterol 0mg

# 2 - Spicy Roasted Carrots

**Preparation time: 10 minutes**

**Cooking time: 30 minutes**

**Serves: 4**

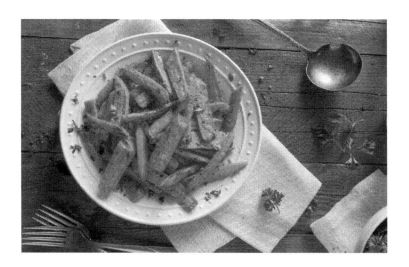

## Ingredients:

- 1lb carrots, peeled & cut into small slices
- ¼ tsp chili powder
- ¼ tsp cinnamon
- ½ tsp ground coriander
- ½ tsp paprika
- ½ tsp cumin
- 2 tsp olive oil
- Pepper
- Salt

## Directions:

- Preheat the oven to 400F.
- In a mixing bowl, add carrots and remaining ingredients and toss until well coated.
- Spread carrot slices onto a baking sheet and roast in preheated oven for 25-30 minutes. Stir halfway through.
- Serve and enjoy.

## Nutritional value (amount per serving):

- Calories 69
- Fat 2.5g
- Carbohydrates 11.6g
- Sugar 5.6g
- Protein 1.1g
- Cholesterol 0mg

# 3 - Roasted Garlic Turmeric Cauliflower

**Preparation time: 10 minutes**

**Cooking time: 40 minutes**

**Serves: 4**

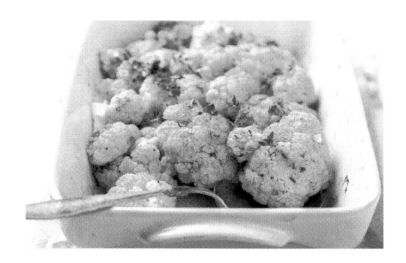

## Ingredients:

- 1 medium cauliflower, cut into florets
- 2 tbsp fresh parsley, chopped
- 3 tbsp olive oil
- ½ tsp garlic powder
- ¾ tsp turmeric powder
- 1 head of garlic, roughly chopped
- Pepper
- Salt

## Directions:

- Preheat the oven to 375F.
- In a large bowl, toss cauliflower florets with oil, garlic powder, turmeric, garlic, pepper, and salt.
- Spread cauliflower florets onto a parchment-lined baking sheet and roast in preheated oven for 40 minutes. Stir halfway through.
- Garlic with parsley and serve.

## Nutritional value (amount per serving):

- Calories 129
- Fat 10.7g
- Carbohydrates 8.3g
- Sugar 3.6g
- Protein 3g
- Cholesterol 0mg

# 4 - Sauteed Kale with Garlic & Lemon

**Preparation time: 10 minutes**

**Cooking time: 5 minutes**

**Serves: 4**

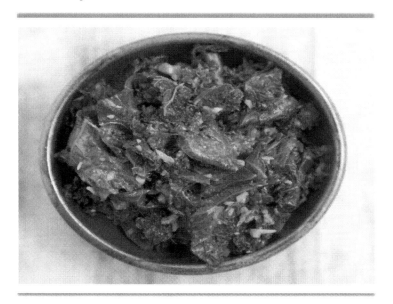

## Ingredients:

- 1 bunch kale, chopped
- 2 garlic cloves, chopped
- 2 tsp olive oil
- ½ lemon juice
- Pepper
- Salt

## Directions:

- Heat oil in a large pan over medium heat.
- Add garlic, kale, pepper, and salt and sauté until kale is wilted, about 2-4 minutes. Turn off the heat.
- Add lemon juice and toss well.
- Serve and enjoy.

## Nutritional value (amount per serving):

- Calories 34
- Fat 2.4g
- Carbohydrates 2.9g
- Sugar 0.1g
- Protein 0.8g
- Cholesterol 0mg

# 5 - Cauliflower Rice Pilaf

## Preparation time: 10 minutes

## Cooking time: 5 minutes

## Serves: 2

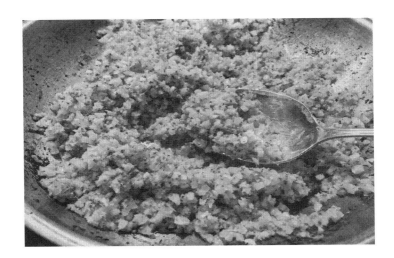

## Ingredients:

- 1lb cauliflower rice
- 1 tbsp lemon juice
- ½ tsp garlic, minced
- ¼ cup onion, chopped
- ½ cup cilantro, chopped
- 2 tbsp olive oil
- 1 tsp turmeric
- Pepper
- Salt

## Directions:

- Heat olive oil in a pan over medium heat.
- Add garlic and onion to the pan and sauté for minute.
- Add turmeric and sauté for 30 seconds.
- Add cauliflower rice and cook over medium-high heat for 5 minutes or until rice is cooked.
- Add cilantro, lemon juice, pepper, and salt and stir well.
- Serve and enjoy.

## Nutritional value (amount per serving):

- Calories 261
- Fat 18.3g
- Carbohydrates 17.8g
- Sugar 9.9g
- Protein 9.3g
- Cholesterol 0mg

# 6 - Grilled Asparagus with Lemon & Parmesan

**Preparation time: 10 minutes**

**Cooking time: 5 minutes**

**Serves: 4**

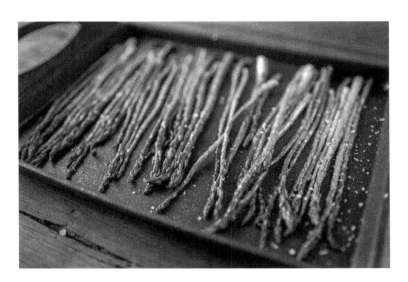

## Ingredients:

- 1lb asparagus; cut the woody ends
- 3 tbsp Parmesan cheese, shredded
- ½ lemon juice
- 1 tbsp olive oil
- ½ lemon zest
- Pepper
- Salt

## Directions:

- Preheat the grill to high heat.
- In a large bowl, toss asparagus with oil, pepper, and salt.
- Arrange asparagus onto a hot grill and cook for 3-5 minutes.
- Transfer grilled asparagus onto a serving platter and top with lemon juice, lemon zest, and shredded Parmesan cheese.
- Serve and enjoy.

## Nutritional value (amount per serving):

- Calories 71
- Fat 4.8g
- Carbohydrates 4.8g
- Sugar 2.3g
- Protein 4.2g
- Cholesterol 4mg

# 7 - Balsamic Roasted Brussels sprouts

**Preparation time: 10 minutes**

**Cooking time: 25 minutes**

**Serves: 4**

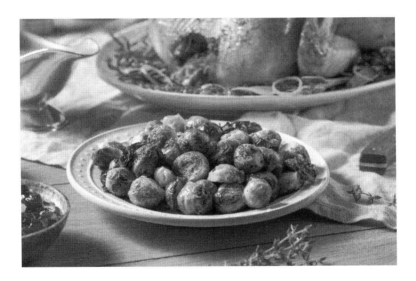

## Ingredients:

- 1½lbs Brussels sprouts, cut in half
- 2 garlic cloves, minced
- 2 tbsp olive oil
- 2 tbsp balsamic vinegar
- Pepper
- Salt

## Directions:

- Preheat the oven to 400F.
- In a bowl, toss Brussels sprouts with garlic, oil, vinegar, pepper, and salt.
- Spread Brussels sprouts onto a baking sheet and roast in preheated oven for 20-25 minutes.
- Serve and enjoy.

**Nutritional value (amount per serving):**

- Calories 137
- Fat 7.6g
- Carbohydrates 16.1g
- Sugar 3.7g
- Protein 5.9g
- Cholesterol 0mg

# 8 - Garlic & Herb Roasted Potatoes

**Preparation time: 10 minutes**

**Cooking time: 35 minutes**

**Serves: 4**

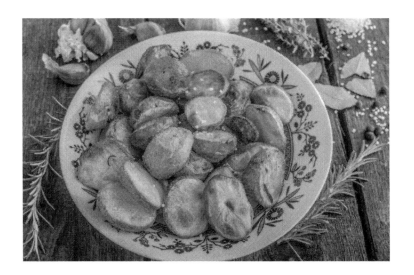

## Ingredients:

- 2lbs baby potatoes, cut in half
- 1 tsp dried parsley
- 1 tsp dried dill
- 2 tbsp olive oil
- 4 garlic cloves, minced
- Pepper
- Salt

## Directions:

- Preheat the oven to 400F.
- In a mixing bowl, toss baby potatoes with parsley, dill, oil, garlic, pepper, and salt until well coated.
- Spread baby potatoes onto a baking sheet and roast in preheated oven for 35 minutes. Stir halfway through.
- Serve and enjoy.

## Nutritional value (amount per serving):

- Calories 197
- Fat 7.3g
- Carbohydrates 29.4g
- Sugar 0g
- Protein 6.1g
- Cholesterol 0mg

# 9 - Beet & Orange Salad with Walnuts

**Preparation time: 10 minutes**

**Cooking time: 40 minutes**

**Serves: 6**

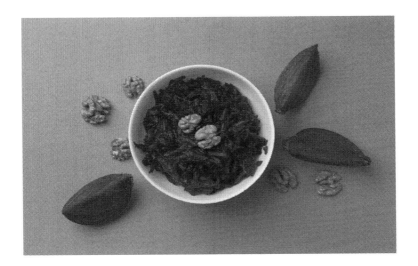

## Ingredients:

- 6 beets, peeled & cut into wedges
- ½ cup feta cheese, crumbled
- ½ cup walnuts, toasted & chopped
- 3 oranges, peeled & cut into segments
- 2 cups baby arugula
- 2 tbsp olive oil
- For dressing:
- 4 tbsp olive oil
- 1 tbsp orange juice

- 1 tbsp honey
- 2 tbsp white wine vinegar
- Pepper
- Salt

## Directions:

- Preheat the oven to 400F.
- Add beets to the baking dish and drizzle with olive oil. Cover and bake for 40 minutes.
- Remove from oven and set aside.
- Add arugula, oranges, and beets into the large bowl.
- In a small bowl, whisk together all dressing ingredients.
- Pour dressing over salad and toss well.
- Top the salad with crumbled cheese and walnuts.
- Serve and enjoy.

## Nutritional value (amount per serving):

- Calories 319
- Fat 23.2g
- Carbohydrates 25.8g
- Sugar 20.4g
- Protein 7g
- Cholesterol 11mg

# 10 - Mashed Sweet Potatoes with Cinnamon

**Preparation time: 10 minutes**

**Cooking time: 15 minutes**

**Serves: 6**

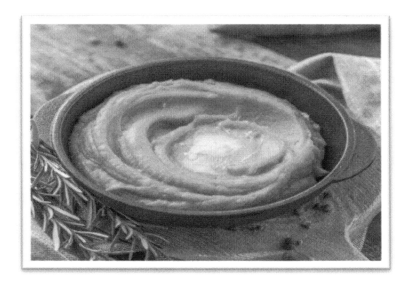

## Ingredients:

- 4lbs sweet potatoes, peeled & cut into 1-inch cubes
- ¼ cup unsweetened almond milk
- 3 tbsp coconut oil
- 1 tsp vanilla extract
- ½ tsp nutmeg
- ½ tsp ginger powder

- 1 tsp cinnamon
- 3 tbsp maple syrup
- 1 tsp salt

**Directions:**

- Add sweet potatoes to the large pot with water and salt. Simmer over medium heat for 15-20 minutes or until tender. Drain sweet potatoes.
- Return sweet potatoes to the same pot and mash with a potato masher.
- Add almond milk, coconut oil, vanilla, nutmeg, ginger powder, cinnamon, and maple syrup and mix until well combined.
- Serve and enjoy.

**Nutritional value (amount per serving):**

- Calories 448
- Fat 7.6g
- Carbohydrates 91.7g
- Sugar 7.6g
- Protein 4.7g
- Cholesterol 0mg

# 11 - Grilled Zucchini with Herbed Yogurt Sauce

**Preparation time: 10 minutes**

**Cooking time: 5 minutes**

**Serves: 2**

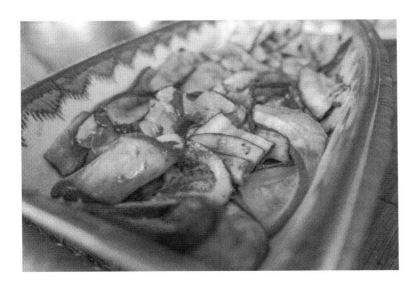

## Ingredients:

- 4 zucchini, cut into slices
- 2 tbsp avocado oil
- Pepper
- Salt
- For yogurt sauce:
- 1 tsp dry dill
- 1 garlic clove, minced

- 1/3 cup plain yogurt
- Salt

## Directions:

- In a bowl, toss zucchini slices with avocado oil, pepper, and salt.
- Arrange zucchini slices onto a preheated grill and cook for 2-3 minutes on each side.
- For sauce: in a small bowl, mix together yogurt, dill, garlic, and salt.
- Serve grilled zucchini slices with yogurt sauce.

## Nutritional value (amount per serving):

- Calories 114
- Fat 3g
- Carbohydrates 17.6g
- Sugar 9.7g
- Protein 7.4g
- Cholesterol 2mg

# 12 - Summer Squash & Tomato Gratin

**Preparation time: 10 minutes**

**Cooking time: 25 minutes**

**Serves: 6**

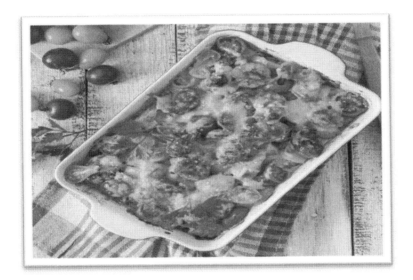

## Ingredients:

- 2 large tomatoes, sliced
- 2 yellow squash, sliced into coins
- ½ cup wholewheat breadcrumbs
- 1 cup Gruyere cheese, shredded
- 1 tsp Italian seasoning
- 1 bell pepper, diced
- 2 shallots, sliced
- Pepper

- Salt

## Directions:

- Preheat the oven to 400F.
- Arrange squash slices into the 9x13-inch baking dish. Season with Italian seasoning, pepper, and salt.
- Sprinkle a small amount of shredded cheese and breadcrumbs over squash slices.
- Layer the tomatoes on top of the squash slices. Repeat with sprinkling Italian seasoning, pepper, salt, cheese, and breadcrumbs.
- Sprinkle shallots and bell pepper on top of tomatoes. Top with remaining Italian seasoning, pepper, salt, cheese, and breadcrumbs.
- Bake in preheated oven for 25 minutes.
- Serve and enjoy.

## Nutritional Value (amount per serving):

- Calories 128
- Fat 6.5g
- Carbohydrates 13.2g
- Sugar 4g
- Protein 8.2g
- Cholesterol 20mg

# 13 - Quinoa Salad with Roasted Vegetables

**Preparation time: 10 minutes**

**Cooking time: 30 minutes**

**Serves: 4**

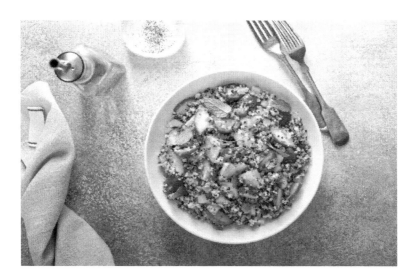

## Ingredients:

- 2 cups cooked quinoa
- 2 garlic cloves, crushed
- ½ tsp Italian seasoning
- ¼ cup onions, diced
- ¼ cup bell peppers, chopped
- ¼ cup cherry tomatoes, sliced in half
- ¼ cup mushroom, sliced

- ½ cup zucchini, diced
- ½ cup yellow squash, diced
- 2 tbsp olive oil
- ½ tsp pepper
- ½ tsp salt

**Directions:**

- Preheat the oven to 400F.
- In a mixing bowl, toss vegetables with oil, Italian seasoning, garlic, pepper, and salt.
- Spread vegetables onto a baking sheet and roast in preheated oven for 30 minutes.
- Add cooked quinoa to the large bowl. Add roasted vegetables to the quinoa.
- Mix well and serve.

**Nutritional value (amount per serving):**

- Calories 390
- Fat 12.5g
- Carbohydrates 58g
- Sugar 1.6g
- Protein 12.9g
- Cholesterol 0mg

# 14 - Greek-style Roasted Eggplant & Peppers

**Preparation time: 10 minutes**

**Cooking time: 30 minutes**

**Serves: 4**

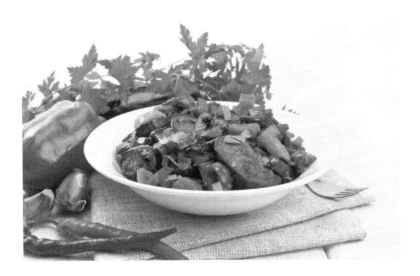

## Ingredients:

- 1 large eggplant, cut into chunks
- 1 large tomato, sliced
- 2 red bell pepper, cut into chunks
- 1 medium onion, sliced
- 2 tbsp apple cider vinegar
- 3 tbsp olive oil
- 2 tbsp parsley, minced

- Pepper
- Salt

## Directions:

- Heat oil in a large pan over medium-high heat.
- Add onion and sauté for a couple of minutes.
- Add eggplant and bell peppers and sauté for 5 minutes.
- Add parsley, garlic, tomato, pepper, and salt, and cook for 2-3 minutes more.
- Transfer the eggplant and bell pepper mixture to the baking pan and roast in preheated oven at 350F for 30 minutes. Remove from oven and allow to cool completely.
- Add vinegar and mix everything well.
- Serve and enjoy.

## Nutritional value (amount per serving):

- Calories 154
- Fat 11g
- Carbohydrates 15.8g
- Sugar 8.9g
- Protein 2.5g
- Cholesterol 0mg

# 15 - Gingered Carrot & Sweet Potato Mash

**Preparation time: 10 minutes**

**Cooking time: 20 minutes**

**Serves: 8**

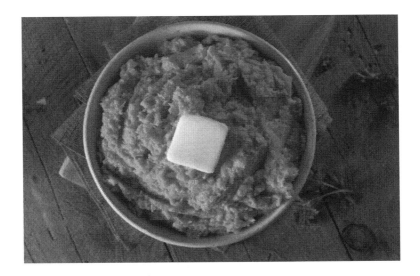

## Ingredients:

- 4 medium carrots, peeled & chopped
- 2 medium sweet potatoes, peeled & chopped
- ½ tsp turmeric
- ¼ tsp ground ginger
- 2 garlic cloves, minced
- 2 tbsp coconut oil, melted
- Salt

## Directions:

- Add sweet potatoes and carrots to the large pot. Cover with water and bring to boil over high heat.
- Turn heat to medium-high and continue to cook for 10-15 minutes or until carrots and sweet potatoes are tender.
- Drain carrots and sweet potatoes and return to the pot.
- Add boiled carrots and sweet potatoes into the food processor along with turmeric, ginger, garlic, coconut oil, and salt and process until smooth.
- Serve and enjoy.

## Nutritional value (amount per serving):

- Calories 88
- Fat 3.5g
- Carbohydrates 13.8g
- Sugar 1.7g
- Protein 0.9g
- Cholesterol 0mg

# Chapter 7 – Dessert Recipes

## The Place of the Dessert dish in the Anti-Inflammatory Diet

The desserts within an anti-inflammatory diet are meant to fulfill your sweet tooth without sacrificing your health goals. Natural sweeteners like maple syrup, honey, and fruit are frequently used in their preparation because of the health benefits they provide. These options have a lesser effect on blood sugar levels and a lower glycemic index than refined sugar. Desserts often have fruits with antioxidants in them. Apples, berries, citrus fruits, and pomegranates are examples of fruits that contain high levels of vitamins, fiber, and antioxidants. These fruits fight inflammation and give extra health benefits.

Desserts in a diet that helps reduce inflammation can have good fats like nuts, seeds, and avocados. These fats make you feel full, help desserts taste smooth, and have anti-inflammatory properties. Making desserts at home allows for better control over ingredients and customization. By preparing desserts from scratch, you can choose healthier alternatives, adjust sweetness levels, and incorporate anti-inflammatory ingredients according to your preferences.

Dessert dishes in an anti-inflammatory diet are best enjoyed in moderation. While they may contain healthier ingredients, it's important to maintain balance in your overall diet and not rely heavily on desserts. Opting for fruit-based desserts, smoothies, yogurt parfaits, or desserts with minimal added sugars can help satisfy sweet cravings while promoting anti-inflammatory benefits.

The place of dessert dishes in an anti-inflammatory diet is to provide a sense of balance and enjoyment. While the focus is on incorporating healthier ingredients, it's also important to satisfy cravings and indulge in treats from time to time. By choosing anti-inflammatory dessert options, you can still enjoy the flavors and pleasures of dessert while supporting your health goals. These desserts offer a healthier option for satisfying your sweet tooth without sacrificing your health.

# 1 - Mixed Berry Parfait with Coconut Yogurt

**Preparation time: 5 minutes**

**Cooking time: 5 minutes**

**Serve: 1**

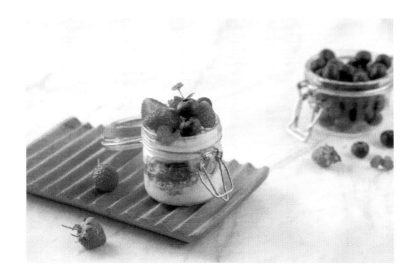

## Ingredients:

- ½ cup mixed berries
- ½ tbsp ground flaxseeds
- ½ banana, sliced
- ½ cup granola
- ½ cup coconut yogurt

## Directions:

- Add granola and ground flaxseeds into the serving glass, then top with banana slices and yogurt.
- Top with mixed berries and serve.

## Nutritional value (amount per serving):

- Calories 311
- Fat 32.8g
- Carbohydrates 95.6g
- Sugar 43.8g
- Protein 22.6g
- Cholesterol 0mg

# 2 - Chia Seed Pudding with Fresh Fruits

**Preparation time: 5 minutes**

**Cooking time: 5 minutes**

**Serves: 4**

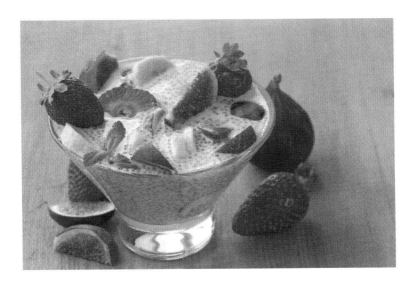

## Ingredients:

- ½ cup chia seeds
- ¾ cup plain yogurt
- 1 & 2/3 cups unsweetened almond milk
- 2 tbsp honey
- 2 cups fresh fruits

## Directions:

- In a medium bowl, mix together almond milk and chia seeds and set aside for 5 minutes.
- Add honey and yogurt to the chia seed mixture and whisk until well combined.
- Pour chia pudding into the four serving jars, cover and place in refrigerator for 8 hours.
- Top each jar with fruits and serve.

**Nutritional value (amount per serving):**

- Calories 153
- Fat 3.6g
- Carbohydrates 27.2g
- Sugar 19.8g
- Protein 4.7g
- Cholesterol 3mg

# 3 - Baked Apples with Cinnamon & Walnuts

**Preparation time: 10 minutes**

**Cooking time: 20 minutes**

**Serves: 6**

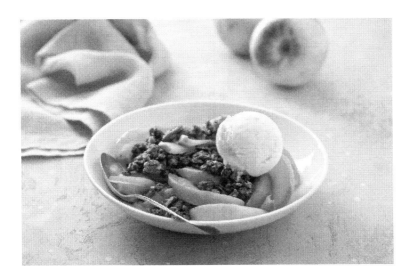

## Ingredients:

- 6 large apples, cored & sliced
- 1 tbsp ground cinnamon
- ½ cup walnuts, chopped
- ½ cup honey
- 4 tbsp coconut oil, melted

## Directions:

- Preheat the oven to 350F.
- In a baking dish, mix together melted coconut oil, cinnamon, honey, and walnuts.
- Add apple slices and mix everything well.
- Bake in preheated oven for 20-25 minutes.
- Serve and enjoy.

## Nutritional value (amount per serving):

- Calories 347
- Fat 15.6g
- Carbohydrates 56g
- Sugar 46.5g
- Protein 3.2g
- Cholesterol 0mg

# 4 - Avocado Chocolate Mousse

**Preparation time: 5 minutes**

**Cooking time: 5 minutes**

**Serves: 4**

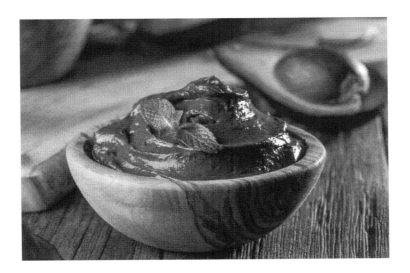

## Ingredients:

- 3 avocados; scoop out the flesh
- 2 tbsp maple syrup
- ¼ cup unsweetened almond milk
- 3 tbsp unsweetened cocoa powder
- Pinch of salt

## Directions:

- Add avocado, maple syrup, almond milk, cocoa powder, and salt into the blender and blend until smooth.
- Divide the mousse into the serving glasses and store in the fridge until ready to serve.

## Nutritional value (amount per serving):

- Calories 345
- Fat 30.2g
- Carbohydrates 22g
- Sugar 6.8g
- Protein 3.7g
- Cholesterol 0mg

# 5 - Mango Coconut Ice Cream

**Preparation time: 10 minutes**

**Cooking time: 5 minutes**

**Serves: 6**

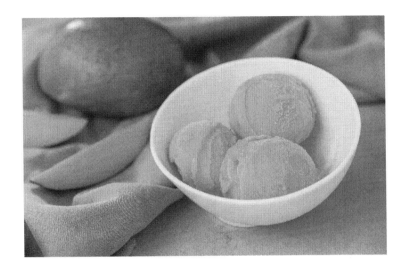

## Ingredients:

- 4 cups frozen mango chunks
- 2 tbsp maple syrup
- 1 cup full-fat coconut milk
- Pinch of salt

## Directions:

- Add frozen mango chunks, maple syrup, coconut milk, and salt into the blender and blend until smooth and creamy.

- Serve immediately and enjoy.

## Nutritional value (amount per serving):

- Calories 163
- Fat 8.4g
- Carbohydrates 22.3g
- Sugar 19.7g
- Protein 1.6g
- Cholesterol 0mg

# 6 - Blueberry Almond Crisp

**Preparation time: 10 minutes**

**Cooking Time: 40 minutes**

**Serve: 6**

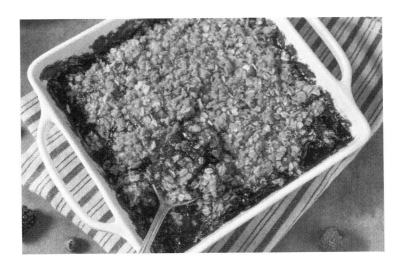

## Ingredients:

- 4 cups blueberries
- ½ cup almond meal
- ¼ cup maple syrup
- ¼ cup olive oil
- ½ cup pecans, chopped
- 1 cup old-fashioned oats
- ½ tsp salt

## Directions:

- Preheat the oven to 350F.
- Add blueberries into the 8x8-inch baking dish.
- In a bowl, mix together oats, maple syrup, olive oil, almond meal, pecans, and salt.
- Sprinkle the oats mixture evenly over the blueberries.
- Bake in preheated oven for 35-40 minutes.
- Serve and enjoy.

## Nutritional value (amount per serving):

- Calories 266
- Fat 14.6g
- Carbohydrates 33.7g
- Sugar 18.1g
- Protein 4.2g
- Cholesterol 0mg

# 7 - Banana Oat Cookies

**Preparation time: 10 minutes**

**Cooking time: 15 minutes**

**Serves: 18**

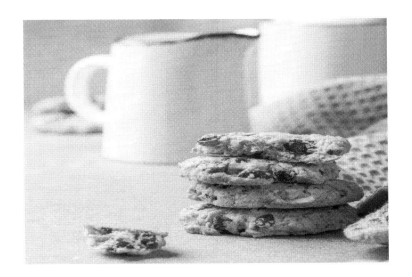

## Ingredients:

- 1 egg
- 1 ¼ cups mashed banana
- ½ cup dried cranberries
- 1 tsp cinnamon
- 1 ½ cups quick oats
- 1 tsp vanilla
- 2 tbsp honey
- ¼ tsp sea salt

## Directions:

- Preheat the oven to 350F.
- In a mixing bowl, mix together mashed bananas, vanilla, egg, and honey.
- Add oats, cranberries, cinnamon, and salt and stir until well combined.
- Make equally shaped dough balls from the oats mixture and arrange them onto a parchment-lined baking sheet.
- Slightly press down each dough ball with your fingers to create a circle-shaped cookie.
- Bake cookies in preheated oven for 12-15 minutes. Remove cookies from oven and allow to cool completely.
- Serve and enjoy.

## Nutritional value (amount per serving):

- Calories 48
- Fat 0.7g
- Carbohydrates 9.4g
- Sugar 3.4g
- Protein 1.3g
- Cholesterol 9mg

# 8 - Lemon Poppy Seed Energy Balls

**Preparation time: 10 minutes**

**Cooking time: 10 minutes**

**Serves: 10**

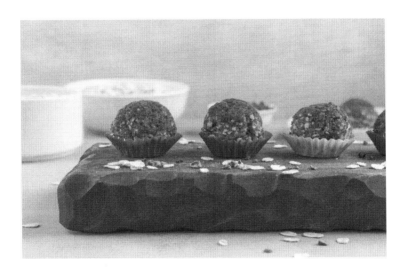

## Ingredients:

- 1 tbsp poppy seeds
- 2 tbsp lemon juice
- 1 cup almond flour
- 1 lemon zest, grated
- 1 tbsp coconut butter, melted
- ¼ cup maple syrup
- ¼ cup creamy cashew butter
- 1 cup shredded sweetened coconut
- 1 cup oat flour

## Directions:

- Add all ingredients into the food processor and process until smooth and well combined.
- Make equally-shaped of balls from the mixture and place onto a plate.
- Serve and enjoy.

## Nutritional value (amount per serving):

- Calories 90
- Fat 3.7g
- Carbohydrates 13.1g
- Sugar 5.4g
- Protein 1.7g
- Cholesterol 0mg

# 9 - Pumpkin Spice Baked Oatmeal Bars

**Preparation time: 10 minutes**

**Cooking time: 30 minutes**

**Serves: 4**

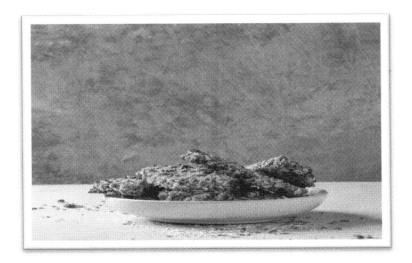

## Ingredients:

- 1 ½ cups oats
- 2 tbsp ground flaxseed
- ½ tsp pumpkin pie spice
- 1/3 cup unsweetened almond milk
- 1/3 cup pumpkin puree
- 2 tbsp maple syrup
- 1 tsp cinnamon
- 1 tsp baking powder
- ¼ cup coconut sugar

## Directions:

- Add oats and remaining ingredients into a large mixing bowl and mix until well-combined.
- Pour the oats mixture into the greased 9x9-inch baking dish and spread evenly.
- Bake at 350F for 30 minutes.
- Remove from oven and let it cool completely.
- Cut into pieces and serve.

## Nutritional value (amount per serving):

- Calories 175
- Fat 3.5g
- Carbohydrates 31.5g
- Sugar 7g
- Protein 5g
- Cholesterol 0mg

# 10 - Raspberry Chia Jam Bars

**Preparation time: 10 minutes**

**Cooking time: 30 minutes**

**Serves: 16**

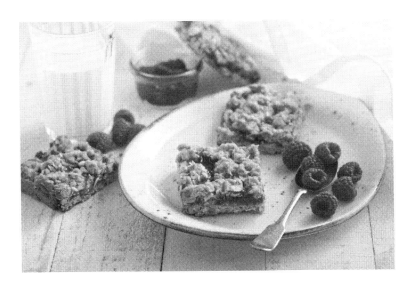

## Ingredients:

- 2 chia eggs
- 1 cup raspberry chia jam
- ¼ cup Erythritol
- 1 tsp baking powder
- 3 tbsp coconut oil
- 2 tbsp almond butter
- ¾ cup ground almonds
- 1 cup oat flour

- ¼ tsp salt

## Directions:

- Preheat the oven to 350F.
- In a mixing bowl, mix together the oat flour, sweetener, baking powder, ground almonds, and salt.
- Add almond butter, chia eggs, and coconut oil and mix until well combined.
- Transfer ¾ of the oat flour mixture into a parchment-lined 8-inch cake pan. Spread the mixture evenly and press down using a spatula.
- Bake in preheated oven for 10 minutes.
- Remove from oven and spread the jam on top. Sprinkle the remaining oat mixture over the jam layer and bake for 20 minutes more.
- Remove from oven and let it cool completely.
- Cut into pieces and serve.

## Nutritional value (amount per serving):

- Calories 136
- Fat 6.8g
- Carbohydrates 20.2g
- Sugar 15.1g
- Protein 2.8g
- Cholesterol 0mg

# 11 - Almond Flour Banana Bread

**Preparation time: 10 minutes**

**Cooking time: 55 minutes**

**Serves: 15**

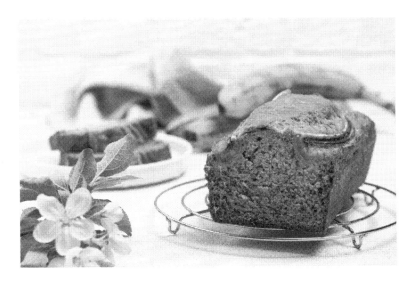

## Ingredients:

- 2 eggs
- 3 ripe bananas, mashed
- 2½ cups almond flour
- 1 tsp baking powder
- 1 tsp baking soda
- 1 tsp cinnamon
- 1 tsp vanilla extract
- ¼ cup coconut oil

- ¼ cup maple syrup
- ¼ tsp salt

## Directions:

- Preheat the oven to 325F.
- Spray a 9x5-inch loaf pan with cooking spray and set aside.
- In a mixing bowl, mix together eggs, mashed bananas, vanilla, coconut oil, and maple syrup until well combined.
- Stir in the almond flour, baking powder, baking soda, cinnamon, and salt until combined.
- Pour batter into the prepared loaf pan and bake in preheated oven for 50-55 minutes. Remove from the oven and allow to cool for 10 minutes.
- Slice and serve.

## Nutritional value (amount per serving):

- Calories 76
- Fat 4.3g
- Carbohydrates 9.3g
- Sugar 6.1g
- Protein 1g
- Cholesterol 22mg

# 12 - Coconut Flour Pancakes with Berries

**Preparation time: 10 minutes**

**Cooking time: 10 minutes**

**Serves: 6**

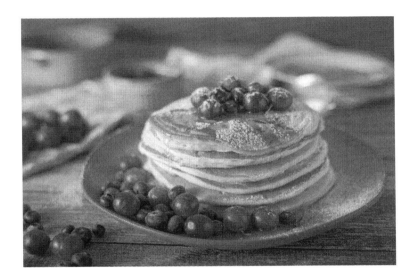

## Ingredients:

- 3 eggs
- 1 tsp vanilla
- 1 tsp baking powder
- 2 tbsp maple syrup
- 2 tbsp olive oil
- ¼ cup coconut flour
- 1/8 tsp sea salt

## Directions:

- In a mixing bowl, whisk together eggs, vanilla, baking powder, maple syrup, oil, coconut flour, and salt until well combined.
- Spray a large pan with cooking spray and heat over medium-low heat.
- Spoon 3 tablespoons of the batter onto a hot pan and cook for 4-5 minutes, turn pancake and cook for 4 minutes. Repeat with the remaining batter.
- Serve pancakes with fresh berries.

## Nutritional value (amount per serving):

- Calories 112
- Fat 7.4g
- Carbohydrates 8.5g
- Sugar 4.2g
- Protein 3.4g
- Cholesterol 82mg

# 13 - Cocoa Almond Truffles

**Preparation time: 10 minutes**

**Cooking time: 5 minutes**

**Serves: 8**

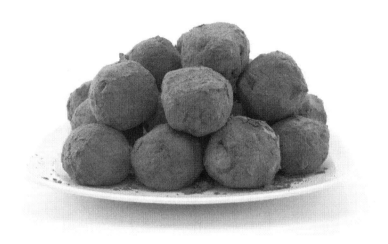

## Ingredients:

- 1 cup almonds
- 2 tbsp water
- ½ tsp vanilla extract
- ¼ cup cocoa powder
- 10 Medjool dates, pitted
- Pinch of salt

## Directions:

- Add almonds, water, vanilla, 2 tablespoons of cocoa powder, dates, and salt into the food processor and process until the mixture forms a sticky dough ball.
- Make equally-shaped balls from the mixture and place onto a parchment-lined plate. Place in fridge for 30 minutes.
- Add remaining cocoa powder in a small bowl then roll each ball in cocoa powder to coat completely.
- Serve and enjoy.

## Nutritional value (amount per serving):

- Calories 250
- Fat 6.3g
- Carbohydrates 49.1g
- Sugar 36.8g
- Protein 4.2g
- Cholesterol 0mg

# 14 - Matcha Green Tea Popsicles

**Preparation time: 10 minutes**

**Cooking time: 5 minutes**

**Serves: 6**

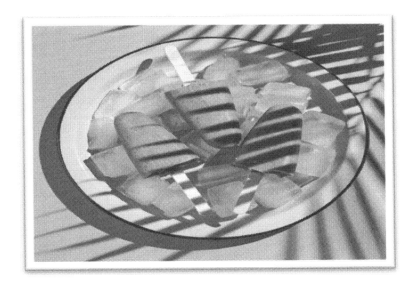

## Ingredients:

- 1 tbsp matcha green tea powder
- 1 tbsp vanilla extract
- ½ cup Medjool dates, pitted
- ½ cup water
- 1/3 cup cashews, soaked for 4 hours & drained
- 1 cup coconut cream

## Directions:

- Add all ingredients into a blender and blend until smooth.
- Pour blended mixture into the popsicle molds and place in the freezer for overnight.
- Serve and enjoy.

## Nutritional value (amount per serving):

- Calories 142
- Fat 9.2g
- Carbohydrates 5g
- Sugar 2g
- Protein 2.1g
- Cholesterol 0mg

# 15 - Baked Pear with Honey & Cinnamon

**Preparation time: 10 minutes**

**Cooking time: 30 minutes**

**Serves: 4**

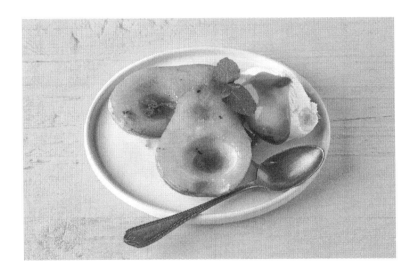

## Ingredients:

- 4 medium pears, peeled, cut in half & core scooped out
- ½ tsp vanilla extract
- ½ tsp cinnamon
- 2 tbsp coconut oil
- 3 tbsp honey

## Directions:

- Preheat the oven to 400F.
- Arrange pears face down into the baking dish.
- In a small bowl, mix together honey, vanilla, oil, and cinnamon.
- Spoon honey mixture over pears.
- Bake pears in preheated oven for 30 minutes. Remove from oven and allow to cool for 5 minutes.
- Serve and enjoy.

## Nutritional value (amount per serving):

- Calories 205
- Fat 7g
- Carbohydrates 38.6g
- Sugar 29.2g
- Protein 0.7g
- Cholesterol 0mg

# Chapter 8-Meal Planning and Tips

## Anti-Inflammatory Meal Plan for Two Week

### Week One Meal Plan:

- **Monday**
- Breakfast: Overnight Chia Pudding
- Lunch: Quinoa & Chickpea Salad with Roasted Vegetables
- Dinner: Baked Salmon with Lemon & Dill

- **Tuesday**
- Breakfast: Vegetable Omelet
- Lunch: Greek-style Roasted Eggplant & Peppers
- Dinner: Turmeric Chicken Stir-Fry

- **Wednesday**
- Breakfast: Quinoa Breakfast Bowl
- Lunch: Roasted Sweet Potato & Kale Salad with Maple Dijon Dressing
- Dinner: Quinoa Stuffed Bell Peppers

- **Thursday**
- Breakfast: Banana Walnut Muffins
- Lunch: Quinoa Stuffed Bell Peppers
- Dinner: Mediterranean Baked Chicken

- **Friday**
- Breakfast: Avocado Toast with Smoked Salmon
- Lunch: Summer Squash & Tomato Gratin
- Dinner: Moroccan Chickpea Stew

- **Saturday**
- Breakfast: Blueberry Oatmeal Breakfast Bars
- Lunch: Arugula & Pomegranate Salad with Toasted Pecans
- Dinner: Zucchini Noodles with Turkey Meatballs

- **Sunday**
- Breakfast: Sweet Potato & Kale Breakfast Skillet
- Lunch: Quinoa Salad with Roasted Vegetables
- Dinner: Sweet Potato Black Bean Enchiladas

# Week Two Meal Plan:

- **Monday**
- Breakfast: Healthy Scrambled Eggs
- Lunch: Quinoa & Spinach Stuffed Portobello Mushrooms
- Dinner: Eggplant & Chickpea Tagine

- **Tuesday**
- Breakfast: Almond Butter Banana Wrap
- Lunch: Sauteed Kale with Garlic & Lemon
- Dinner: Baked Cod with Herb Crust

- **Wednesday**
- Breakfast: Veggie Breakfast Burrito
- Lunch: Gingered Carrot & Sweet Potato Mash
- Dinner: Sweet Potato Black Bean Enchiladas

- **Thursday**
- Breakfast: Buckwheat Pancakes with Fresh Berries
- Lunch: Grilled Shrimp & Vegetable Skewers
- Dinner: Baked Cod with Herb Crust

- **Friday**
- Breakfast: Mushroom & Spinach Egg Muffins
- Lunch: Kale & Quinoa Salad with Lemon Tahini Dressing
- Dinner: Cauliflower Fried Rice

- **Saturday**
- Breakfast: Quinoa Banana Bread
- Lunch: Greek Salad with Feta & Olives
- Dinner: Mediterranean Baked Chicken

- **Sunday**
- Breakfast: Vegetable Omelet
- Lunch: Roasted Vegetable Salad with Turmeric Dressing
- Dinner: Baked Salmon with Lemon & Dill

# Tips for Eating out on the Anti-Inflammatory Diet

- ➢ Focus on whole, unprocessed foods.

- ➢ Make sure to eat different types of colorful fruit and vegetables with your meal

- ➢ Choose anti-inflammatory fats like olive oil, avocados, and nuts.

- ➢ Incorporate fatty fish rich in Omega-3 fatty acids, such as salmon or sardines.

- ➢ Opt for lean sources of protein like poultry, fish, beans, and lentils.

- ➢ Minimize or avoid processed and sugary foods.

- ➢ Reduce your consumption of red and processed meats during your diet.

- ➢ Use herbs and spices like turmeric, ginger, and garlic to add flavor and anti-inflammatory benefits.

- ➢ Drink lots of water during the day to keep your body hydrated.

- ➢ Consume wholegrains like quinoa, brown rice, and oats.

- ➢ Include nuts and seeds like almonds, walnuts, flaxseeds, and chia seeds for healthy fats and fiber.

- ➢ Avoid or limit refined carbohydrates like white bread and pasta.

- ➢ Opt for low-glycemic index foods that have a minimal impact on blood sugar levels.

- ➢ Prioritize fiber-rich foods like vegetables, fruits, wholegrains, and legumes.

- ➢ Incorporate probiotic-rich foods like yogurt or fermented vegetables to support gut health.

- ➢ Minimize or avoid processed vegetable oils high in Omega-6 fatty acids, such as soybean or corn oil.

- ➢ Stay away from artificial additives, preservatives, and sweeteners.

- ➢ Drink less alcohol because it can cause inflammation.

- ➢ Remember to pay attention to how much you eat to keep a healthy weight.

- ➢ Cook at home more often to have control over ingredients and cooking methods.

- ➢ Try doing activities like meditation, deep breathing, or yoga to help manage stress.

- ➢ Engage in regular physical activity to reduce inflammation and promote overall well-being.

- ➢ Get enough sleep each night to support proper recovery and immune function.

- ➢ Be aware of food sensitivities or allergies and avoid triggering foods.

- ➢ Choose organic produce and pasture-raised or organic animal products whenever possible.

- Read food labels and avoid products with added sugars, hydrogenated oils, and artificial ingredients.

- Experiment with plant-based meals by incorporating more fruits, vegetables, and legumes.

- Try herbal teas like green tea, chamomile, or ginger tea for their anti-inflammatory properties.

- Limit your intake of high-sodium foods to help manage inflammation and blood pressure.

- Practice portion control with high-calorie foods to maintain a healthy weight.

- Choose natural sweeteners like honey or maple syrup in moderation instead of refined sugar.

- Incorporate cruciferous vegetables like broccoli, cauliflower, and Brussels sprouts for their anti-inflammatory benefits.

- Snack on fresh fruits, vegetables, or homemade snacks instead of processed snacks.

- Use cooking methods like grilling, baking, steaming, or sautéing instead of deep frying.

- Stay hydrated with herbal infusions, lemon water, or flavored water without added sugars.

- Incorporate anti-inflammatory spices like cinnamon, cayenne pepper, or turmeric into your meals.

- Limit or avoid high-fat and fried foods that can promote inflammation.

- Keep a food journal to track how certain foods affect your body and identify potential triggers.

- Cook with antioxidant-rich ingredients like berries, dark chocolate, and colorful spices.

- Practice moderation with caffeine intake, as excessive consumption can contribute to inflammation.

- Incorporate natural sources of antioxidants, such as green leafy vegetables and berries, into your diet.

- Avoid or limit processed snack foods like chips, cookies, and candy.

- Choose low-fat or non-fat dairy products like yogurt, milk, or cheese.

- Include fermented foods like sauerkraut, kimchi, or kefir for their probiotic benefits.

- Opt for gluten-free grains like quinoa, buckwheat, or amaranth if you have gluten sensitivity.

- Minimize or eliminate intake of artificial trans-fats found in processed and fried foods.

- Incorporate prebiotic-rich foods like onions, garlic, asparagus, and bananas to support a healthy gut microbiome.

- Experiment with alternative sweeteners like stevia or monk fruit extract instead of refined sugar.

- Choose organic, grass-fed, or pasture-raised meats and poultry to minimize exposure to antibiotics and hormones.

- Include anti-inflammatory herbs like basil, rosemary, thyme, and parsley in your cooking.

- Practice portion control by using smaller plates and bowls to help manage calorie intake.

- Avoid or minimize consumption of processed and sugary condiments like ketchup, barbecue sauce, and salad dressings.

- Be mindful of your Omega-6 to Omega-3 fatty acid ratio by reducing your intake of processed and fried foods high in Omega-6 fats.

- Include plenty of garlic and onions in your meals, as they contain compounds that have anti-inflammatory properties.

- Experiment with plant-based protein sources like tofu, tempeh, or seitan.

- Limit consumption of high-fructose corn syrup found in many processed foods and beverages.

- Choose dark chocolate with a high percentage of cocoa for its antioxidant and anti-inflammatory properties.

- Reduce exposure to environmental toxins by choosing organic produce and using non-toxic household and personal care products.

➢ Practice mindful grocery shopping by reading labels and choosing products with minimal ingredients and no artificial additives.

➢ Enjoy a variety of herbs and herbal teas known for their anti-inflammatory effects, such as chamomile, ginger, or Echinacea.

➢ Engage in regular physical activity like walking, cycling, or swimming to support overall health and reduce inflammation.

➢ Practice portion control with high-calorie foods and use mindful eating techniques to listen to your body's hunger and fullness cues.

➢ Seek support and accountability by joining an anti-inflammatory diet support group or partnering up with a friend or family member.

➢ Be patient and consistent with your dietary changes, as it may take time for your body to respond and for inflammation to decrease.

➢ Avoid or limit the consumption of processed breakfast cereals high in added sugars and artificial ingredients.

➢ Incorporate seaweed, such as nori or kelp, into your diet for its rich mineral content and potential anti-inflammatory benefits.

➢ Use a variety of cooking methods, such as steaming, baking, grilling, or stir-frying, to preserve nutrients and add flavor to your meals.

➢ Practice intuitive eating by paying attention to your body's hunger and fullness cues and eating in response to physical hunger rather than emotional cues.

➢ Seek guidance from a registered dietitian or healthcare professional who specializes in anti-inflammatory nutrition for personalized advice and recommendations tailored to your specific needs and health goals.

# Conclusion

The anti-inflammatory diet is recognized as a strong tool for improving health and lowering inflammation in the body. It stresses the consumption of whole, nutrient-dense foods while minimizing or avoiding pro-inflammatory ingredients. The scientific research and studies performed on the anti-inflammatory diet provide significant proof for its usefulness in lowering inflammation markers, controlling chronic conditions, and boosting general well-being.

One of the most important things to come out of the study is that sticking to an anti-inflammatory diet can make inflammation signs better and disease activity goes down. For example, a randomized controlled cross-over experiment called the Anti-Inflammatory Diet in Rheumatoid Arthritis (ADIRA) study protocol examined the effect of an anti-inflammatory diet on disease activity and quality of life in rheumatoid arthritis patients. The study hoped to discover whether the anti-inflammatory diet could improve symptoms and overall well-being in people with this condition. The results of the study are anticipated to shed light on the potential benefits of the diet in managing inflammation and enhancing the quality of life for those with rheumatoid arthritis. Additionally, the Multiethnic Cohort Study studied the relationship between commitment to an anti-inflammatory diet and mortality risk. The study followed a big cohort of men and women over an extended time to assess the effect of the diet on long-term health results. The data showed that greater adherence to an anti-inflammatory diet was linked with a reduced chance of mortality in both men and women. This shows the ability of the diet to improve longevity and overall health.

The anti-inflammatory diet offers numerous health benefits beyond inflammation decrease. It has been shown to improve cardiovascular health by lowering the chances of heart disease and improving lipid levels. The focus on whole, plant-based foods, lean proteins, and healthy fats promotes heart-healthy decisions and supports optimal cardiovascular performance. Additionally, diet has a good effect on metabolic health and weight control. By supporting the consumption of nutrient-dense foods and minimizing processed and high-sugar choices, it helps regulate blood sugar levels, improve insulin sensitivity, and reduce the risk of getting type 2 diabetes. The addition of high-fiber foods such as fruits, veggies, and wholegrains adds to satiety, aids in weight control, and supports healthy gut bacteria.

Furthermore, the anti-inflammatory diet has been linked to better gut health. The consumption of fiber-rich foods, probiotics, and prebiotics helps feed the gut microbiota, promoting a wide and healthy microbial community. A healthy gut microbiome is linked with lower inflammation, better digestion, increased nutrient intake, and stronger immune function.

Mental health and brain performance are also strongly affected by the anti-inflammatory diet. Chronic inflammation has been involved in different mental health problems, including sadness and anxiety. By reducing inflammation, the diet may have a positive effect on mood and mental well-being. Furthermore, the addition of Omega-3 fatty acids from sources like fatty fish, flaxseeds, and walnuts benefits brain health and cognitive function.

Meal planning and preparation play a crucial part in properly following an anti-inflammatory diet. By planning, making a shopping list, and cooking meals at home, people have better control over the ingredients used and serving sizes. This allows for the inclusion of fresh, nutrient-dense foods and the avoidance of processed or pro-inflammatory ingredients found in pre-packaged meals or fast food. In addition to food planning, following other healthy habits and lifestyle factors can further improve the benefits of the anti-inflammatory diet. Regular physical activity not only aids in weight management but also helps reduce inflammation and improves overall cardiovascular health. Stress management methods, such as mindfulness meditation or yoga, can add to a healthy reaction to stress and lower inflammation levels. Adequate sleep and staying hydrated are also important for supporting general health and lowering inflammation in the body. It is important to recognize that the anti-inflammatory diet is not a one-size-fits-all method. Each person may have unique dietary needs, tastes, and sensitivities.

Consulting with a healthcare worker or certified dietitian can provide personalized advice and ensure that the anti-inflammatory diet is suitable and tailored to individual needs.

In conclusion, the anti-inflammatory diet offers a strong method for improving general health and lowering inflammation in the body. By focusing on whole, nutrient-dense foods and minimizing pro-inflammatory ingredients, people can support their well-being, control chronic conditions, and promote longevity. An anti-inflammatory diet is one of the healthiest ways to improve the quality of your life. It combines scientific study, incorporating anti-inflammatory foods, and making healthy lifestyle choices.

## Leave the Review

As an independent author with a small marketing budget, reviews are my livelihood on Amazon. If you enjoyed this book, I'd really appreciate it if you leave your honest feedback on Amazon. I love hearing from my readers, and I personally read every single review.

## Thank you

# Reference Page

Abdallah, J., Assaf, S., Das, A., & Hirani, V. (2023). Effects of anti-inflammatory dietary patterns on non-alcoholic fatty liver disease: a systematic literature review. *European Journal of Nutrition, 62*(4), 1563–1578. https://doi.org/10.1007/s00394-023-03085-0

Barhum, L. (2022). 5 signs of inflammation. *Verywell Health.* https://www.verywellhealth.com/signs-of-inflammation-4580526

Binu, S. (2021, August 10). Inflammation: Types, Causes, Symptoms And Treatment. *Netmeds.* https://www.netmeds.com/health-library/post/inflammation-types-causes-symptoms-and-treatment

CDN, J. L. M. R. (2023, February 6). 12 things you need to know about the Anti-Inflammatory Diet. *Good Housekeeping.* https://www.goodhousekeeping.com/health/diet-nutrition/g4487/anti-inflammatory-diet/

Fand, A. L. M. R. L. (2022). Anti-Inflammatory salads. *Eat Love Gut Health.* https://angelalagonutrition.com/anti-inflammatory-salads/

Fisher, L. (2023, May 26). 5 Anti-Inflammatory breakfast ideas to start your morning on a healthy note. *Real Simple.* https://www.realsimple.com/health/nutrition-diet/anti-inflammatory-breakfast#:~:text=The%20Benefits%20of%20Eating%20an%20Anti%2DInflammatory%20Breakfast&text=Both%20dieticians%20agree%20that%20breakfast,lifestyle%20and%20helps%20fight%20inflammation.

*Five Principles For An Anti-inflammatory Diet | Piedmont Healthcare.* (n.d.). https://www.piedmont.org/living-better/the-anti-inflammatory-diet

Graffouillère, L., Deschasaux, M., Mariotti, F., Neufcourt, L., Shivappa, N., Hébert, J. R., Wirth, M. D., Latino-Martel, P., Hercberg, S., Galan, P., Julia, C., Kesse-Guyot, E., & Touvier, M. (2016). Prospective association between the Dietary Inflammatory Index and mortality: modulation by antioxidant supplementation in the SU.VI.MAX randomized controlled trial. *The American Journal of Clinical Nutrition, 103*(3), 878–885. https://doi.org/10.3945/ajcn.115.126243

Kaluza, J., Håkansson, N., Harris, H. R., Orsini, N., Michaëlsson, K., & Wolk, A. (2018). Influence of anti-inflammatory diet and smoking on mortality and survival in men and women: two prospective cohort studies. *Journal of Internal Medicine, 285*(1), 75–91. https://doi.org/10.1111/joim.12823

Lawler, M. (2023, February 24). *Anti-Inflammatory Diet: Diet: how it works, benefits, foods, and more.* EverydayHealth.com. https://www.everydayhealth.com/diet-nutrition/diet/anti-inflammatory-diet-benefits-food-list-tips/

Professional, C. C. M. (n.d.). *inflammation*. Cleveland Clinic. https://my.clevelandclinic.org/health/symptoms/216 60-inflammation#:~:text=Inflammation%20is%20an%2 0essential%20part,may%20lead%20to%20chronic%2 0inflammation

Rd, J. K. M. (2020, April 8). *15 healthy staples you should always have on hand*. Healthline. https://www.healthline.com/nutrition/healthy-staples#2.-Nuts,-seeds,-and-their-butters

Singh, A. S. M. a. P., MD. (2021). Key benefits of the Anti-Inflammatory Diet — Dr. Amar Singh and Dr. Poonam Singh. *Dr. Amar Singh and Dr. Poonam Singh.* https://www.drsinghs.com/blog/anti-inflammatory-diet

Winkvist, A., Bärebring, L., Gjertsson, I., Ellegård, L., & Lindqvist, H. M. (2018). A randomized controlled cross-over trial investigating the effect of anti-inflammatory diet on disease activity and quality of life in rheumatoid arthritis: the Anti-inflammatory Diet In Rheumatoid Arthritis (ADIRA) study protocol. *Nutrition Journal*, *17*(1). https://doi.org/10.1186/s12937-018-0354-x

Zwickey, H., Horgan, A., Hanes, D., Schiffke, H. C., Moore, A., Wahbeh, H., Jordan, J., Ojeda, L., McMurry, M. P., Elmer, P. J., & Purnell, J. Q. (2019).

239

Made in United States
Troutdale, OR
12/30/2023

16555296R00133